As the major cause of vision impairment among older adults, macular degeneration affects the lives of millions. Yet among the public, little is known about this disease and its impact on visual functioning. This very readable and informative book goes far in providing older persons and their families with the knowledge they need to cope with macular degeneration. Covered are the range of preventive, therapeutic, and rehabilitative interventions that are available. Most important, the book conveys the essential message that, while a cure for macular degeneration has not yet been found, much can be done in some cases to arrest the progress of the disease and in all cases to help the patient function independently and with quality of life in spite of the disease.

—Dr. Barbara Silverstone
President and CEO
Lighthouse International

LIVING WELL WITH MACULAR DEGENERATION

PRACTICAL TIPS AND ESSENTIAL INFORMATION

DR. BRUCE P. ROSENTHAL AND KATE KELLY

NEW AMERICAN LIBRARY

New American Library
Published by New American Library, a division of
Penguin Putnam Inc., 375 Hudson Street, New York, New York 10014, U.S.A.
Penguin Books Ltd, 27 Wrights Lane, London W8 5TZ, England
Penguin Books Australia Ltd, Ringwood, Victoria, Australia
Penguin Books Canada Ltd, 10 Alcorn Avenue, Toronto, Ontario, Canada M4V 3B2
Penguin Books (N.Z.) Ltd, 182–190 Wairau Road, Auckland 10, New Zealand

Penguin Books Ltd, Registered Offices: Harmondsworth, Middlesex, England

Published by New American Library, a division of Penguin Putnam Inc.

First Printing, April 2001
10 9 8 7 6 5 4 3 2 1

LIBRARY OF CONGRESS CATALOGING-IN-PUBLICATION DATA:
Rosenthal, Bruce P.
    Living well with macular degeneration : practical tips and essential information /
Bruce P. Rosenthal and Kate Kelly.
        p.   cm.
    Includes index.
    ISBN 0-451-20264-3 (alk. paper)
    1. Retinal degeneration—Popular works.   I. Kelly, Kate.   II. Title.

    RE661.D3 R675 2001
    617.7'35—dc21

                                                      00-066843

Set in New Caledonia
Designed by Eve L. Kirch

Printed in the United States of America

CONTENTS

Introduction   1
A Word from Dr. Bob Thompson   7
A Word from Dr. David Guyer   13

Part I. When Vision Begins to Change

1. The Truth About Macular Degeneration   17
2. What AMD Does to the Eye   24
3. The Eye Exam   35
4. Treatment Options   53
5. The Risk Factors of AMD and What You
   Can Do About Them   67
6. Carrots and Beyond: Helping Yourself Nutritionally   75

Part II. Extra Vision When You Need It

7. Maximizing Sight: Simple Ways to See Better   89
8. Making the Best Use of Low-Vision Devices   103

Part III. Practical Advice for Living Well

9.	Basic Principles	131
10.	Your Home Environment	141
11.	Simple Systems for Daily Tasks	151
12.	Can I Still Drive?	163
13.	Out and About	194
14.	Advice for Others	212
	Conclusion	220
	Appendix: What Is Covered by Insurance and What Is Not	223
	Glossary	225
	Resources	232
	Acknowledgments	257
	Index	260

INTRODUCTION

During my college years when I was at home visiting, one of the family tasks I performed regularly was driving my grandmother on errands or bringing her to our house for family visits. This was a new relationship for us. Ruth had always been extremely independent and loved driving, but she could no longer operate a car—she was losing her vision. She loved to cook and garden, read and play bridge, and she was a major baseball fan. She and my grandfather went to the local baseball games, and they loved watching national games on television.

Because of her worsening vision, she had had to make changes in the way she lived. When I visited the summer after my grandfather died, I often found her listening to a book on tape instead of holding her usual paperback in her hand. Her oven dial had 350 marked in red nail polish to make it easier for her to set a basic temperature. My mother bought a big magnifying glass that attached to the television screen so she could still watch baseball games. Fortunately, long before her vision problems became a hindrance to her, she had moved to an apartment with a beautiful common area where she spent a great deal of her time socializing with a newly developed circle of friends.

At age twenty-one, I didn't really understand what was happening to my grandmother other than that she was "losing her vision." My impression was that it was just one of those things that happens to some older people. If the doctor ever actually gave a name to the disease when he discussed her condition with her, I was never made aware of it. The doctor did, however, mention a likely cause—smoking, which we now know is one of many possible causes of macular degeneration.

Sixteen years after her death, I still pull out recipes in her handwriting, oversized letters written in dark black ink. At the time I received them, they were just "Ruth's recipes," but today I see them in an entirely new light, because I realize that while reading normal print was difficult for her, she could still follow a recipe if the writing was large enough and black enough.

Recently my mother was diagnosed with macular degeneration, and I now have a name for the condition that affected my grandmother. When my mother first told me, her vision had barely begun to change. She mentioned it briefly during the intermission of a play, and the topic was raised more as a warning to me than as information about her: "Start taking antioxidant vitamins." (Vitamins may help slow the onset of the disease.) The curtain went up, and what with one thing and another, she was on her way back to Colorado before I realized we had never had a full discussion about what "macular degeneration" meant.

I soon found that knowing the name for this disease was only moderately helpful. Wanting to find out what was ahead for my mother, I began looking for information. At night, at a time when surfing the Internet was quite new, I would run searches for "macular degeneration." Each time I came up with very little. Eventually, I found a Web site for a certain style of low-vision device. The aeronautics engineer-turned-inventor, who created it, Ed Bettinardi, began answering my questions about macular degeneration. He, too, had become interested in the field when his mother developed the disease. I slowly began learning what having macular degeneration involved.

I am a writer by profession, and the books I undertake often grow out of personal curiosity about a subject that I want to know more about. Macular degeneration certainly fit that criterion. If I couldn't find helpful information for my mom, then other people were almost certainly similarly stymied. I felt there was a need for a book on the topic. What was this disease called age-related macular degeneration, or AMD? What should we expect? What could we do?

I changed the direction of my pursuit. Instead of seeking out information, I started looking for an expert to help me write the book. As I talked to various people, the name that kept recurring was that of Dr. Bruce Rosenthal, Chief of Low Vision Programs at Lighthouse International in New York City.

When we met at his offices, I found an optimistic, caring individual who always had an upbeat story to tell about one of his patients. From our initial conversation, I learned that as a specialist in low vision, Dr. Rosenthal may have the perfect job. Though there are no pharmaceutical cures for AMD, no helpful surgery, and the latest laser treatments benefit only a limited few, there are a wide variety of helpful low-vision devices (with more on the way) that help the visually impaired see their world again. Dr. Rosenthal is among the fortunate few in this field who can promise hope to the discouraged by providing them with a "new way of seeing."

Dr. Rosenthal first became interested in low vision (then called "subnormal" vision) while he was teaching at the State

University of New York College of Optometry in New York City. In 1974, he joined the staff of what is now known as Lighthouse International and became one of their low-vision clinicians and part of the low-vision education team. Working with the top experts in eye care, Dr. Rosenthal began expanding his knowledge of the field.

Since that time Dr. Rosenthal has been instrumental in helping to establish the clinical low-vision programs at the College of Optometry as well as at other low-vision services in New York City. Currently, in his position at Lighthouse International, a world-renowned vision rehabilitation organization and resource for information on vision impairment and rehabilitation, he maintains an active practice and travels internationally speaking on issues concerning low vision.

When I proposed to him the idea of coauthoring a book, I was met with an enthusiastic reaction. "Both patients and their families need a way to learn about AMD," he said, and we set to work. Through Dr. Rosenthal I have met caring and concerned medical professionals who are working hard to devise answers for those with AMD. In addition, I have met delightful, hopeful, positive patients, who have been very willing to share with me the challenges of the disease (and there are many) as well as how they have avoided letting the diagnosis get them down.

Together we will share with you (and your family, I hope, for they want to understand what is happening, too) all we know about macular degeneration.

How to Use This Book

Following this introduction are two additional introductions by experts in the field of macular degeneration. Dr. Bob Thompson, Chairman of the AMD Alliance International, writes with warmth and humor about his hard-won adjustment to his own diagnosis of macular degeneration. Dr. David Guyer, one of the foremost experts in the field, shares hopeful news about the latest medical search.

Living Well with Macular Degeneration is divided into three parts. The first section, "When Vision Begins to Change," explains what you need to know about macular degeneration and provides the latest information available about treatment and ways to possibly keep the disease from progressing.

Part Two, "Extra Vision When You Need It," is a rundown on the glasses, magnifiers, and technological inventions that have been created to amplify what you can see.

In Part Three, "Practical Advice for Living Well," you'll find guidance on going about your daily life. There's a great deal you can do for yourself to make life more convenient and fun. There's also a chapter that provides advice to others. If you find that your neighbor starts speaking more loudly to you when she hears you have macular degeneration, you'll realize why people need a primer on what it means to have low vision!

When your eye-care doctor tells you nothing more can be done, keep in mind that your doctor is referring only to medical treatment for the disease itself. A lot more can be done through vision-rehabilitation services that help you function better by making the best use possible of your remaining vision and acquiring skills in the activities of daily living. Unfortunately vision-rehabilitation services are not widely available. There is no Medicare coverage for vision-rehabilitation therapists and limited coverage for low-vision clinicians. (Fortunately, a bill is now before Congress to partially corrrect this situation.) The Resource section in the back of this book lists organizations, toll-free information numbers, Web sites, catalogs, and pamphlets that can point you in the right direction.

Finally, at times this book will read as if you have barely any vision with AMD, and at other times we're cheerfully discussing people with the disease who are still driving. You may rightly wonder, "What's going on here?"

Every case of AMD is different. Some diagnoses are made early enough that a person may have very mild vision loss; others are diagnosed only after loss is quite profound. Even then the AMD experience varies widely. Some people who can no longer see to read a book see well enough to drive, and many who see well enough to read can no longer drive.

Take the advice that applies to your situation, and keep the book handy. Come back to it later, when there's something else you'd like to know.

Kate Kelly
April 2001

A WORD FROM DR. BOB THOMPSON

"I am sorry. There is nothing more I can do for you. . . ."
There I was, back in 1992, happily chugging along, saving lives in my chosen profession as a general practitioner in North Yorkshire, England. During that summer, I noticed a strange, persistent visual distortion in my right eye, coupled with difficulty in adjusting to dark from light; noticeably, the dashboard instruments in my car were hard to read. Naturally, as a doctor, I paid little heed to such trivia. Yet within two years, my cherished, hard-earned career was gone, and I was registered legally blind. Failing to appreciate in myself what would have rung alarm bells in my brain had it been one of my patients, I had failed to recognize the early symptoms of age-related macular degeneration (AMD). At 48, I was unusually young to develop this disease.

I had "wet" AMD, the less common but more severe form. It will be of small surprise to learn that the other type of AMD is termed "dry." The wet type tends to progress more rapidly and involves growth of unwanted new blood vessels, like a membrane, under the central retina or macula. As the membrane grows, it leaks and may bleed, ultimately disrupting the health of the macula and often leading to quite sudden and profound central visual impairment. Dry AMD tends to progress much more slowly; it involves a gradual deterioration of central vision due to the steady functional decline in the cells of the macula. Dry AMD accounts for around 90% of all AMD. Although wet AMD constitutes the remaining 10%, it accounts for around 90% of AMD folk who are legally blind.

In 1992, and even now in 2000, there was no treatment for dry AMD, and the only conventional treatment for wet AMD was photocoagulation: using a "hot" laser beam to destroy the growing membrane before it caused permanent damage. Unfortunately, the hot laser beam destroys healthy as well as diseased tissue, so it is suitable for only a tiny minority of cases, where the membrane is far enough from the center of the macula. Laser treatment failed in my case. Within weeks my other eye developed a membrane, this time right under the center of the macula, rendering it unsuitable for laser treatment. At this point, things started to get really bad. I faced numerous visits to a powerless ophthalmologist, endless tests, the brain-numbing shock of realizing that my most precious faculty would soon be seriously compromised.

How can you prepare for such an awful inevitability? For me, it was a dry-mouthed, damp-palmed, heart-palpitating wait. It cannot be—maybe it won't happen, I told myself. Appalled family members, friends, and colleagues rallied around me, desperate to help. I have been intoned over by kindly clerics. I've experienced faith healing, aromatherapy, reflexology, homeopathy, and radiotherapy. Finally, I was savagely impaled by an unbelievably zealous acupuncturist.

Notwithstanding any of those treatments, within a few weeks, late one Friday afternoon, with a shimmer and a brief final shake, my remaining "good" macula gave up the unequal struggle and lifted off the back of my eye. My vision, already distorted, was now shrouded, as though I were looking through dense net curtains.

Thus began life without the sight that I had taken for granted. I had to learn to face each day robbed of the ability to read; unable to recognize simple objects and the faces of family and friends; incapable of doing simple tasks like unplugging a lamp or writing a letter, watching TV, attending the movies or theater, appreciating the beauty of my surroundings and, perhaps the worst, the final apotheosis of loss of independence, driving a car.

The psychological trauma is hard to describe, and even harder to imagine until such a disaster happens to you. When my second eye failed, I almost felt relieved; the miserable anticipation was almost worse than the event. At least now I could stop worrying about it. My adjustment was essentially a process of bereavement; after all, one is mourning a very real loss. Different people experience varying degrees of shock, disbelief, anger, and denial, and without help, they often slide slowly into depression. Many of us follow this path, and many stay there, in despair.

A natural reaction is to begin a desperate search for a cure. I was no exception, and as a computer-literate doctor, I was well placed to trawl the ophthalmological world for anyone who was on the verge of a "breakthrough." Anyone who could put an end to this nightmare and "put it back like it was."

I just wanted my sight back!

But there was no one—lots of interesting research ideas and programs, but nothing near fruition. Wiser and sadder, I turned my attention to ways and means of restoring as much normality to everyday living as I possible could, arguing that I had to live today, tomorrow, and the next day. Sitting around waiting for a cure, I could grow seriously old with an impoverished quality of life.

A visit to Baltimore, Maryland, brought me into contact with an innovative piece of "hi-tech" low-vision technology. Designed and produced by a team from the Wilmer Institute, Johns Hopkins University, it was a portable head-mounted device incorporating video technology together with an image-intensification system borrowed from NASA. With fired-up enthusiasm, I realized that this could be the beginning of a new line in low-vision aids. This device could lead to increasingly sophisticated, highly portable technology capable of restoring mobility with enhanced imaging and, thus, represent a significant step toward improving the quality of my life.

Since returning from Baltimore five years ago, kitted out with the new technology and looking like a refugee from the planet Zog, I have kept up with developments and, on the whole, been proved right. There are a variety of hi-tech electronic aids on the market, each generation an improvement over the last. They are getting lighter, easier to use with better image quality, cosmetically more acceptable and, most important, cheaper. Together with a variety of more conventional low-tech equipment, they form a vital part of my low-vision aids armory.

The "built environment" (I know! I don't like it either!) is important, too. By careful thought and planning, trial and error, and finally (a last resort) seeking advice, I redesigned the topography and lighting of my house so that I could continue to do my domestic tasks, hobbies, and activities as near-to-normally as possible. I like to cook, so the kitchen was a priority. Abundant, strong, focused halogen spotlights now light work surfaces in colors and patterns that offer high contrast. Utensils are now conveniently placed, and if other members of the family move them, they receive the pain of my withering sarcasm. I serve meals on plain, pastel colored crockery: I got fed up trying to eat patterns! On my piano, a table lamp with a long neon tube provides well-directed diffuse light over a wide area. I read music wearing spectacle frame–mounted binoculars. Areas where I read, using low-vision aids, are adorned with a variety of clip-on lights, and table and floor lamps throw good light over my shoulder onto the reading material. My computer is adapted for speech and reads documents to me. I use an electrostatic "drawing board" device as a computer mouse, enabling me to indulge other hobbies, such as drawing, painting, and photography. I can hand-write letters again and send them directly by fax or e-mail through the computer. The computer also serves as an answering machine and can preset telephone numbers with one click of the mouse. There is little I cannot do that I could do before AMD, except drive. But that is only part of the story.

For the past five years, I have been heavily involved in all aspects of macular disease, keeping abreast of burgeoning areas of research, increasing my understanding of the causes, thoroughly up-to-date on the hunt for treatments, cures, and prevention. Advances are being made all the time, but there is still a long way to go. While never losing sight of a possible future treatment, I'm still very aware that for the vast majority of us the only sensible option is learning to live with AMD.

As I look back over the years, I realize there was a turning point for me, a moment when I knew it was pointless to keep mourning what was gone. It was better to figure out how to make the best of what remained. The problem was not with my eyes, but between my ears—a battle of the mind. Living successfully with AMD begins with motivation, and an understanding that you can do a lot to improve your situation. Adapting may be slow and even painful at times. It took me months to train myself to put my peripheral vision to good functional use. Trial and error brought me to find low-vision aids that best enhanced this new skill.

Accept help and advice wherever you can—from low-vision centers (if they exist near you), from self-help groups, and from books like this one.

"I am sorry. There is nothing more that can be done for you" are useless words that too many of us have heard from our medical attendants in the early stages of our journey through AMD. It isn't true!

> Dr. Bob Thompson
> Chairman, Macular Disease Society (UK)
> Chairman, AMD Alliance International
> April 2001

A WORD FROM DR. DAVID GUYER

NEW TREATMENTS OFFER HOPE FOR
PATIENTS WITH MACULAR DEGENERATION

After years with little progress in the treatment of age-related macular degeneration (AMD), this new century brings with it signs that advancement is at last being made.

The FDA recently approved the drug Visudyne for photo-dynamic therapy. This treatment appears to be effective on a limited basis for some people with wet AMD.

While this is a definite step forward, a great deal of progress still needs to be made. Pharmacological (drug) intervention appears especially promising in the treatment of AMD.

The advantages of drug treatment for macular degeneration are considerable. With drugs, we can avoid the possibility of laser-induced retinal damage. We also may be able to prevent dry AMD from progressing to wet by treating certain cases prophylactically.

Early drug studies for AMD, involving the use of interferon, were discouraging, but now with a better understanding of the angiogenic process (the growth of new blood vessels, which is what occurs in wet AMD), new pharmacological agents are being tried at different stages of the disease.

The processes being explored for use in AMD are similar to those being tried in the treatment of cancer when drugs are administered to try to destroy tumors by cutting off the growth of abnormal blood vessels. Similarly, it is hoped that sight can be preserved by reducing the bleeding of the weak abnormal vessels that occur with wet AMD.

Later in the book, you'll read about anti-VEGF therapy, which is one of the types of antiangiogenic treatments being explored.

Other types of drugs being investigated include metalloproteinase inhibitors—drugs that are designed to halt the enzyme (metalloproteinase) that permits the body to build the unwanted blood vessels that cause wet AMD. Over one hundred patients have been recruited for a clinical trial with results to be announced in the near future.

Another very exciting clinical trial that has just started involves an angiostatic steroid that is given by injection.

These clinical trials—as well as several others that are getting underway—are what we hope will be early steps toward a safe and effective treatment for AMD.

You and your family should keep abreast of progress in the field by following the news and checking related Web sites. In the coming years, we hope for new developments that will benefit patients with this devastating disease.

David Guyer, M.D.
Professor and Chairman
NYU School of Medicine
April 2001

PART I

WHEN VISION BEGINS TO CHANGE

1

The Truth About Macular Degeneration

If you're like most people, you knew very little—or nothing at all—about macular degeneration when your doctor said that you, or someone you love, had signs of the condition.

Though age-related macular degeneration (AMD) is the most common cause of visual loss in the United States and other developed countries, AMD was until recently a disease no one talked about. Few could have identified it as a progressive loss—usually gradual—of central vision. Though most people with AMD retain good peripheral (side) vision, the loss of central vision—the part of the eye that brings in detail—eventually results in difficulty driving, reading, and recognizing faces.

In the past, many people assumed that a gradual worsening of eyesight was just something that happened as people got older.

According to a 1995 survey by the Lighthouse, one in six Americans forty-five years or older (17 percent or 13.5 million) reports some form of vision impairment even when wearing glasses. Based on the most recent figures available from Prevent Blindness America (1990), an estimated 13.2 million Americans age forty and over (15 percent) have signs of macular degeneration. More than 1.2 million (1.4 percent) have serious vision loss from macular degeneration. (Prevent Blindness America is the only organization to have gathered and analyzed the statistics, and the figures gathered primarily concerned Caucasians.) If the current trend continues, over the next thirty-five years the number of people with AMD will double. As people live longer, AMD is becoming a health crisis waiting to happen.

To address the problem, the government is devoting unprecedented amounts of money to research age-related eye problems including macular degeneration. When a person's AMD grows worse, he or she may no longer be able to see well even with prescription eyeglasses, a condition that is now termed "low vision." In 1999, the National Eye Institute unveiled a major campaign about low vision. As a result, more and more people are becoming aware of this epidemic.

Today we know that a drop in visual acuity does not have to be a part of growing older. And we are learning that, even after a diagnosis of macular degeneration, a great deal can be done to preserve the sight you have and make the best use of it. While no cure for AMD currently exists, there are ways for those diagnosed to maintain independent lifestyles, through treatment and rehabilitation options, low-vision devices, and support services.

The body of information on the topic is growing all the time. The more you learn about the condition, the better prepared you'll be to ask questions that will lead to helpful answers. The best place to start is by separating facts from misinformation.

Common Worries

Lack of familiarity breeds undue worry and concern. Here are answers to some of the worries shared by most people:

"I'm afraid I'll go blind."

This is everyone's first—and worst—fear. Studies show that Americans fear losing their sight more than losing any other sense. A person with macular degeneration will notice a worsening of his or her central vision—the part of the eyesight that focuses on details. Though occasionally central vision loss is sudden, most often it progresses slowly. Unless a person has other eye diseases to complicate the situation, he will retain peripheral (side) vision, which provides adequate vision for getting around. Some people who have quite serious central vision loss report that over time they learn to see more with their peripheral vision than they did when the central loss first occurred. In addition, special low-vision devices can refract (re-aim) peripheral vision so that details (reading material, for example) can be seen.

"You say I won't go blind, but my sister has AMD and has been diagnosed as 'legally blind.'"

There's a big difference between legal blindness and total blindness. This is explained later in the book. For the time being, be assured that many people who are designated as legally blind actually have a good deal of vision left, because they still have peripheral (side) vision.

"I won't be able to read."

As you'll learn, there are many ways that will make it possible for you to continue to read with AMD—and, most exciting, better ways are being found every day.

"Once I start using one of those devices, it's all downhill from there."

Low-vision devices make day-to-day tasks easier, and once you realize they make the difference between being able to do something or not, you'll realize that there's nothing "down-hill" about it.

"My daughter says I ought to learn braille."

It is not necessary for someone with macular degeneration to learn braille in order to access the printed word. There are other ways to read or otherwise absorb the information you need. However, braille should not necessarily be discounted. Some people with AMD do learn braille and find it helpful for simple tasks, such as labeling, or for reading, particularly when they can no longer use low-vision devices.

"I'd better be careful about using my eyes now. I don't want to wear them out."

Using your eyes will definitely not wear them out. Keep looking all around you and trying out some of the ways that make seeing everything you want to see easier. Some people with AMD report that over time they are able to teach themselves to see more with their peripheral vision.

"Why don't you just give me stronger glasses?"

This is a frequent plea from those with AMD. Unfortunately, stronger glasses aren't always the solution. Because macular degeneration creates an actual loss of vision, no type of magnification can bring it back. However, low-vision specialists can work with you to harness what vision you have.

Most people with AMD continue to have almost normal vision throughout their lives. Even those who are severely affected retain enough sight to move about independently, using helpful aids called low-vision devices. In *Twilight: Losing Sight, Gaining Insight*, which he refers to as "an autobiography of his eyes," Henry Grunwald, whose eyesight has now deteriorated a great deal, compares what he sees to J. M. W. Turner's misty landscapes. "I do see a hell of a lot," he told a reporter in an interview with the *New York Times*. "I don't see very clearly."

While surgeons must give up operating, and painters may

choose to change their style of painting, people with AMD still run businesses, participate in competitive sports, and keep up on the latest literature.

"It's really not the worst thing that could happen to you," says one woman who has had AMD for twenty years and now has profound central-vision loss in both eyes. "I still cook, I golf, I take public transportation, and I just recently completed a computer course at the local college where I learned how to use all the low-vision programs for the computer, including getting onto the Internet. There's so much available now it's hard to complain."

Taking Charge

Most of us have lived through difficult illnesses experienced by others. We may have taken them to medical appointments for second or third opinions, read through the information they've gathered from organizations, and helped assess what they (or a family member) have learned about the disease on the Internet.

Being diagnosed with macular degeneration calls for the same type of active participation; you need to reach out for all the information you can about the disease. Remember that you're a pioneer. The generation before you accepted that a reduction in vision "just happens" as you get older; some in the medical community still think that way.

With the increase in government spending on AMD, as well as pharmaceutical companies racing to find ways to slow or halt macular degeneration, you're in the midst of an unfolding story. You can stay on top of the developments by following the news headlines, checking Web sites, and following special-interest newsletters. Your doctor has to keep track of a large number of patients with a variety of ills. This disease can be your special focus.

The best way to become knowledgeable about both your particular case and the field in general is to build a team of experts to advise you. You will use various experts at different times, but to begin, here are the possible candidates who may one day be members of your team:

An *ophthalmologist* is a medical doctor who specializes in eye and vision care. He or she can prescribe medicine and is trained to provide the full spectrum of eye care, from prescribing glasses and contact lenses to performing complex and delicate eye surgery. Many ophthalmologists also conduct scientific research into the causes and cures for eye diseases and vision problems, and some have training in low vision.

An *optometrist* examines, diagnoses, treats, and manages diseases and disorders of the eye and related systemic conditions. These doctors also prescribe eyeglasses and contact lenses, and medicines to treat eye diseases. An increasing number are also beginning to specialize in low-vision care. Some optometrists have training in low vision; they assess vision functioning and prescribe low-vision devices and other vision-rehabilitation services.

An *optician* is the person who crafts and fits corrective lenses from prescriptions written by optometrists and ophthalmologists.

A *retinal specialist* (sometimes referred to as a retinologist) is an ophthalmologist who specializes in diseases of the retina. If you've been diagnosed with macular degeneration, you should be examined by a retinal specialist on a regular basis.

Eventually, you may also want to know about other helpful professionals:

A *low-vision specialist* is an ophthalmologist or, most often, an optometrist, who has acquired specialized training in the treatment of low vision.

Other *vision-rehabilitation professionals* offer help in better ways to live with vision impairment through training in how to use low-vision devices, how to move about safely inside and outside the home, how to make workplace adaptations, and how to accomplish a variety of daily tasks, including cooking and general housekeeping. These professionals include certified *orientation and mobility specialists, rehabilitation teachers,* and *low-vision therapists.* They can usually be found in full-service vision rehabilitation agencies.

Occupational therapists and ophthalmic nurses who receive training in the use of low-vision devices may work in partnership with low-vision specialists.

As when selecting any medical "team," you want well-respected, highly recommended professionals. In addition, you want experts who are seeing many cases of macular degeneration. A vision-rehabilitation agency or low-vision specialist offers you the best expertise. If you have to travel a distance to find someone, it's worth the effort. Your vision is at stake.

2

What AMD Does to the Eye

Early symptoms of macular degeneration are often so slight that if only one eye is affected, a person's good eye may be able to compensate. She may not notice any changes at all in the beginning. If symptoms become noticeable, however, it can be alarming, because the vision is distorted. The pole of a traffic light may suddenly appear wavy, or the fine detail in a photograph may fade. Words in the newspaper may look blurred or the letters seem to break up. Some people report seeing a dark or empty area in the center of the field of vision. In most cases, the change in vision is gradual, not dramatic.

"I first noticed a change when I was on an airplane. I was sitting next to the window, and a great deal of light was coming in, even with the shade half-drawn," describes one man. "The flight attendant was in the aisle offering drinks, and when I turned to her, I noticed a small empty spot in my vision. At the time I thought it was from the light, but then over the course of the trip, I kept noticing this blank place in whatever I was trying to see. When I finally got home and went to my ophthalmologist, he diagnosed me with macular degeneration. I didn't know what it was."

To better understand what happens when a person has AMD, an understanding of the eye and the normal changes that take place within it is helpful.

The Structure of the Eye

The eye is a very complex organ, and in order for you to see, all parts of the organ must function well and in unison.

The Optic Nerve. This is a bundle of nerve fibers that carries visual information from the eye to the brain.

The Cornea. This is a clear tissue that covers the front of the eye and helps focus incoming light.

The Iris and the Pupil. As we view ourselves in a mirror, the visible parts of the eye are the colored iris and the central black pupil. The iris regulates the pupil size. Depending on the amount of background light, the iris constricts or dilates to let more or less light into the eye. The black hole is the pupil, and light needs to pass through this opening in order to create vision.

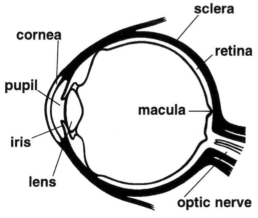

Credit: Lighthouse International

The Lens and Vitreous Gel. Behind the pupil is the clear lens of the eye. The lens focuses light through the vitreous—the clear gel filling the eye—to the retina.

The Retina. This is a very delicate light-sensitive tissue lining the back of the eye. The retina converts light energy that falls on the retina into tiny electrical impulses. It then sends the electrical images via the optic nerve to the brain's visual cortex, where the images are interpreted and a person realizes whose face he sees, what type of bird just flew by, or the number of the bus that is coming down the street. With macular degeneration, however, the pictures that finally make it to the visual cortex and other areas of the brain may be blurry, wavy, distorted, partly missing, or very light. That is because the macula is not functioning properly.

The Macula. Named for the Latin word for "spot," this is the small central portion of the retina, about the size of a nail head. It makes up only 2 percent of the visual field, but it is responsible for central vision, color vision, and fine detail.

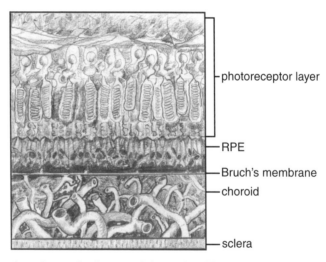

photoreceptor layer

RPE
Bruch's membrane
choroid

sclera

This illustration shows the layers of the retina. The inability of RPE cells to take away waste adversely affects the photoreceptor (light-sensitive) cells, which in turn affects the eye's ability to see clearly.
Credit: Susan Rosenthal

The human eye is often compared to a camera, and if this comparison is extended, then the retina (and macula) is the film. Without a macula that can take in the image through light, tasks such as reading, writing, driving, recognizing faces, cooking, and watching television become very difficult.

The Fovea. The center of the macula is called the fovea. With the highest density of light-receptive cells (photoreceptors), the fovea is the part of the eye that brings in fine detail such as small newsprint.

The Rods and Cones. The all-important light-receptor cells, these form the first layer of cells in the retina. So named because of their shapes, they are responsible for light gathering. Under the rods and cones, which are also called the *photoreceptors*, are the retinal pigment epithelium (RPE) cells. They absorb excess light and dispose of the wastes created by the light-sensing rods and cones. You might think of the RPE cells as the eye's "garbage haulers."

Normal Changes to the Eyes

Like other parts of the human body, the eye deteriorates somewhat over time. By age forty, most people have acquired reading glasses because the older eye has difficulty focusing on items that are close at hand. Other changes occur as time goes on, and they are annoying, but reasonably harmless. Here are a few that occur to almost everyone:

Difficulty adjusting to changes in lighting conditions. As the eye ages, the iris can no longer respond as quickly to changes in light. Most middle-aged and older people are temporarily blinded when entering a darkened movie theater, and a similar delay occurs when stepping out into bright sunlight. The eyes do readjust to the new lighting conditions, but as you age, the process takes more time.

Changes in color perception. The lens in an aging eye yellows a bit and filters out blue light. As a result, certain colors—particularly blacks and dark blues—are difficult to tell apart without bringing the items into bright light.

Some loss of contrast. Vision becomes more difficult under conditions of adverse lighting, and light-colored objects become more difficult to see because of normal changes related to the retina, the lens, and the cornea. Light sensitivity and glare are likewise related to corneal lens and retinal changes.

Floaters. These occur in the vitreous (the jelly-like part of the eye). When bits of this tissue break off and float around, people report seeing "floaters." Many people experience this phenomenon, and though it is annoying at first, most people report that after a short period of time they learn to ignore it.

Other minor conditions such as dryness, burning eyes, fatigue, or a sandy feeling in the eyes can be uncomfortable but can generally be treated.

Changes from Macular Degeneration

To provide vision, the eye automatically adjusts to different levels of light and focuses light through the pupil to the rod and cone receptors of the retina in much the same way that a camera takes in light and images and focuses it on film. Just as a photograph snapped in the dark doesn't come out, if the rods and cones (the photoreceptors) in the eye no longer can accept the light, there is no way to get the image to the macula, and over time you are able to see less and less.

Unlike other types of cells, adult RPE cells (the cells responsible for removing debris from the eye) cannot regenerate. Therefore, when the RPE cells begin to sicken and die from a disease such as macular degeneration, so do the rods and cones they support. As damage to the macula from debris builds up—probably a consequence of a lifetime of wear—central vision fades, and the external world dissolves into an indistinct blur.

To grasp what happens in macular degeneration, think of it as a "rusting" process. The RPE cells are being destroyed, and the resulting debris buildup causes damage to your vision.

While macular degeneration may not be noticeable in its earliest stages, it can produce disabling symptoms as it progresses: blurring of both distance and close vision, an inability to perceive color, a dark or empty area in the center of vision, and a distortion of straight lines.

AMD is actually an umbrella term used to describe a spectrum of changes in the macula. There are two primary forms of the disease: dry AMD and wet AMD. Make sure you know which one you have, because the characteristics and progress of each are different.

Dry Macular Degeneration

The dry form is far more common, affecting 85 to 90 percent of those with the condition. It develops slowly and causes relatively mild vision loss. People with dry AMD notice that reading and other close-vision tasks have become more difficult. This type of AMD is also called atrophic (cells or organs have wasted away and have lost their normal function) macular degeneration.

Often the first sign of dry AMD is drusen, yellow flecks or spots under the retina. These abnormal cellular deposits do not seem to interfere with vision. In fact, hard drusen are fairly common in those under fifty-five, are felt to be relatively harmless, much like age spots on the skin. Hard drusen don't seem to predict the onset of AMD.

In those over fifty-five, large, soft drusen are usually a sign of the disease. Soft drusen can be nearly twice the size of hard drusen. Although the exact role played by soft drusen is still being debated, scientists feel that it may trigger a proliferation of new weaker blood vessels that leak, or in some way contribute to the death of the photoreceptor and RPE cells.

Currently no treatment can reverse the affects of dry AMD, but usually the damage occurs very slowly, so people only gradually notice a blind spot in their central vision, and they don't completely lose their sight. Yet 10 to 15 percent of cases of dry AMD do progress to wet AMD. For that reason, it is essential that you report any changes in your vision to your eye doctor immediately.

Wet Macular Degeneration

Wet macular degeneration is much less common but causes more rapid and severe vision loss. In the wet form of AMD, also called "choroidal neovascularization," there is a buildup of debris that needs to be taken out of your eye, as well as the growth of fragile new blood vessels called choroidal new vessels (CNVs). These weaker, abnormal blood vessels grow (perhaps stimulated by a reduction of nutrients and the slow transport of wastes) and leak blood and fluid under the macula. This interferes with its function by causing distortion under the retina and sometimes by forming scar tissue. This is the form of AMD that most often destroys central vision. Although only 10 percent of people with age-related macular degeneration develop the wet form, it accounts for 90 percent of those who are identified as legally blind.

An early symptom of wet AMD is that straight lines appear wavy. Anything from venetian blinds to a flagpole may suddenly appear to be distorted. This happens because as the newly formed blood vessels leak fluid under the macula, the fluid raises the macula from its normal place at the back of the eye and distorts your vision. Another sign is rapid loss of your central vision. This is different from dry AMD, in which vision loss occurs slowly. As in dry AMD, you may also notice a blind spot.

Cataracts

In many cases AMD is complicated by cataracts, which are common among older people. Cataracts are best described as a clouding of the normally clear lens of the eye. This may range from a very pale opacification that causes little or no interference with vision to dense cloudiness, resulting in marked visual impairment. The rate of progression of cataracts varies from person to person, and their development can vary between the right and left eye in the same person.

Some of the symptoms of cataracts include sensitivity to oncoming headlights of cars, a reduction of vision when wearing sunglasses, the need to shade your eyes when going outdoors in sunlight, glare from fluorescent ceiling lights or bright reading lamps, or difficulty seeing highway signs.

At some point cataracts may become so annoying, or may reduce visual function and visual efficiency so much, that your eye-care professional will discuss with you whether or not the cataracts should be removed through surgery. Though cataract surgery has a 90 to 95 percent success rate, the presence of a preexisting disease such as macular degeneration complicates the situation. When a cataract is covering the eye, doctors are hard pressed to predict, even with testing, how much your vision will improve once the cataract is gone. Unfortunately, there is no clear way to know what the outcome of this type of surgery will be.

Because this condition is much more serious than it is for normal cataract sufferers, ask to be referred to an anterior segment specialist. This is an ophthalmologist who specializes in cataracts. There is some evidence that for people with AMD, the process of removing the cataract and the temporary drop in vitreous pressure causes further hemorrhage and a loss of optic nerve function.

Also keep in mind that any type of surgery carries with it some risk, and you may not get the results you hope for. Sometimes quite serious complications can occur—infection, swelling, or clouding of the cornea, or retinal detachment, to mention just a few. You may even lose more vision in the eye.

New and better methods of correction are being developed. The FDA has just approved a new form of laser cataract surgery (July 2000). A low-energy laser will allow the removal of a cataract through a microincision, making the surgery even less invasive than it is now. The laser produces no clinically significant heat, eliminating heat damage to surrounding tissues and making smaller incisions possible. If you are able to hold out on having cataract surgery until a practitioner in your area offers it, this new type of removal may prove to be a safer one for you.

Peripheral Vision, Visual Acuity, and Functional Vision

Few of us ever think about the types of vision we have. Now you know that you may lose some or all of your central vision. What you will almost certainly maintain is your peripheral vision. This type of vision is best described as those images that reach the part of the retina that surrounds the macula. While this side vision is very important, it is much less clear than macular (central) vision. With side vision we know someone or something is moving in our direction. With central vision we can determine exactly who or what it is. Side vision provides general awareness. Central vision provides analysis.

As you talk to health professionals, you will also hear the terms "visual acuity" and "functional vision." Visual acuity is the ability of the eye to identify detail and objects, and it is this vision that AMD erodes. Visual acuity is what is measured each time you visit the eye doctor and go through the eye chart. These charts are calculated upon the assumption that the individual is seated twenty feet away from the chart. The top number (numerator) refers to the distance of the chart from the patient; the bottom number (denominator) refers to the distance from which a person with perfect vision would be able to read the chart. If your distance vision is recorded as 20/200, you must stand twenty feet away to see the same thing a person with 20/20 vision can see at 200 feet.

Functional vision is the ability to use peripheral vision to get around. People with AMD and no other conditions will maintain functional vision, and some report that over time they learn to absorb more and more information peripherally.

Legal Blindness

Some people with AMD are diagnosed as legally blind, but often that is a long way from being totally blind. Legal blindness is defined as having 20/200 vision in your best eye with correction, or a visual field of 20 degrees or less. This means that with your best eye while wearing glasses or contacts, you see at twenty feet what a normal eye sees at 200 feet. The visual-field measurement is based on the width of the panorama a person sees; a person with a 20-degree visual field is seeing one-ninth of what a normal person sees, which is a full panorama of 180 degrees.

Many people designated as legally blind still see well enough to get around, and they by no means consider themselves to be blind. However, classification of legal blindness does qualify you for certain Social Security and tax benefits as well as certain state services, so take advantage of them. Contact your state's Commission for the Blind to find out more.

Low vision is the term used for a visual impairment that cannot be corrected by standard eyeglasses, contact lenses, medicine, or surgery, and that interferes with the ability to perform everyday activities. It primarily affects people over age sixty-five, and the causes go beyond those related to AMD.

You'll learn more about low vision and the importance of getting a low-vision exam in the next chapter.

3

The Eye Exam

"**I** thought I needed new glasses," Robert says when describing what brought him to the eye doctor when his AMD was first diagnosed. Sometimes people go in for their regular eye exam and are told that they have early signs of macular degeneration. Other people begin to notice some of the following difficulties:

- unable to find personal articles in a familiar environment
- difficulty recognizing faces
- noting that print sometimes looks faded or distorted and that colors often appear faded or washed out
- difficulty judging depth perception on stairs or curbs
- spilling things when reaching across the table because you didn't notice them

Or you may have stopped reading, going through the mail, sewing, or watching TV simply because those activities have become more difficult for you.

If you are told you have early signs of macular degeneration, don't panic. About 80 percent of patients diagnosed with AMD have this early form, and in many, the disease never progresses. Your vision may not worsen noticeably, or it may change at a very slow pace.

However, the diagnosis should be regarded as a wake-up call to take measures to slow the disease. Observational evidence (intelligent opinions formed by researchers through observation, not scientific study) shows that certain lifestyle changes can slow the progress of the disease or even its onset.

But let's go back for a moment. You may find it helpful to know how AMD is detected in the first place.

How AMD Is Detected

Early signs of macular degeneration can generally be spotted by your regular ophthalmologist or optometrist during an annual eye exam. After dilating your eyes, she will check the health of the retina by looking with the ophthalmoscope (a small light) into the back of your eye. The most common early sign is the presence of drusen, the tiny yellow deposits in the retina. Patients may also show signs of altered pigment (changes in the cells of the retina) and perhaps some early atrophy of the layer of cells known as the retinal pigment epithelium (see Chapter 2).

While conducting the examination, your eye-care professional may ask you to look at an Amsler grid. This grid resembles graph paper—some are white on black, others are black on white. You will be asked to cover one eye and stare at a black dot in the center of the grid. While staring at the dot, you may notice that the straight lines in the pattern appear wavy to you. You may notice that some of the lines are missing— signs of wet AMD.

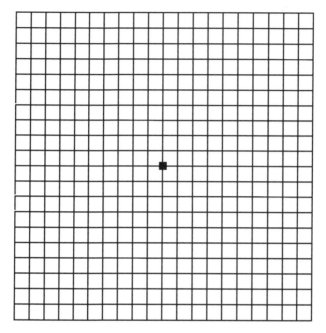

An Amsler grid as it appears to someone with healthy vision.

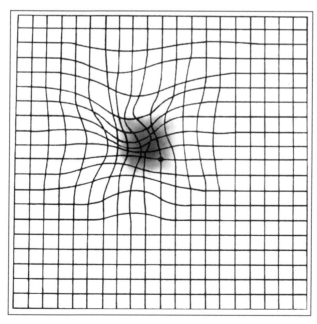

An Amsler grid as it may appear to someone in the early stages of macular degeneration. *Credit: National Eye Institute, National Institutes of Health*

If your doctor suspects you have wet macular degeneration, you will probably be referred to a retinal specialist and have a painless test called fluorescein angiography. In this test a special dye is injected into a vein in the arm. The dye then flows to the blood vessels in the eye, creating a map of the blood vessels in the retina that can then be photographed using a special camera. Depending on the nature and placement of any newly developing weak blood vessels, your doctor can then determine if they can be treated.

Sometimes the fluorescein angiography is not an adequate diagnostic tool because of the particular location of your new blood vessels. If the new growth is under the retina or beneath scar tissue, a computer-enhanced indocyanine green video angiography (ICG) may be recommended. The process for an ICG test is very similar to that of a fluorescein angiography. The dye used in the ICG test contains iodine, so you should tell your doctor if you are allergic to it. These tests have been performed on millions of patients and are extremely safe.

Receiving the News

Sometimes when we receive unexpected news, we find it difficult to accept. "My ophthalmologist told me I had early macular degeneration almost fifteen years ago," says Carl, who now at age seventy-nine has serious vision loss from it. "At the time I just didn't pay much attention to him. I'd never heard of it, and my vision wasn't affected very much by it then, so I didn't even ask any questions."

"I'd never heard of it, and I didn't know what to say or even what to ask," says Helen. "I went home quite upset by it because the one thing I remember him saying was that nothing could be done for it. Then my daughter insisted that we make another appointment and ask questions. We did, but my regular ophthalmologist really wasn't much help. Finally a friend gave me the name of her low-vision specialist, and that was where I finally got the information I needed."

Receiving the news of macular degeneration is never easy. The news is frightening if you know someone who has an advanced case of it, and it's alarming if you've never heard of it before.

Do what Helen did—take someone along with you. An extra pair of ears to listen to what the disease is and what can be done about it will be enormously helpful. In addition, here are some other things you can do:

- Take notes as the doctor talks to you.
- Use a tape recorder to record the conversation so that you can listen again to what was said.
- Ask your doctor to write down instructions for you.
- Ask for printed material about your condition.
- If you have trouble understanding your doctor's answers, ask where you can get more information.
- Other members of your health care team, such as nurses and pharmacists, may be good sources of information. Talk to these people as well.
- Keep asking questions of medical professionals or of personnel from the organizations listed in the Resources section of this book until you are sure that you understand.

If you get a doctor who is overly technical or abrupt and refuses to answer your questions, consider your options. Perhaps another doctor in the same practice would be more helpful. If you can, try to switch to medical personnel who you feel are knowledgeable and willing to help you.

If you are not fully comfortable with the information you are receiving, you have the right to see another doctor. Your doctor should agree to your request and be willing to forward copies of your files to other eye-care professionals. Getting another opinion is respected by any professional who is truly concerned about your well-being, so don't hesitate to ask.

Though greater awareness of macular degeneration is growing in doctor's offices across the country, patients today still report hearing from their regular eye doctor: "There's nothing more I can do for you." Be persistent. Find someone who is knowledgeable. The right person is often a low-vision specialist, but any eye-care professional who is willing to stay on top of new developments in the field can advise you what to do next.

Here is a list of the basic questions to ask your eye-care professional:

- Do I have dry or wet AMD?
- What is the extent of my vision loss, and what other changes might I expect?
- Can you tell how quickly my AMD is progressing?
- Can you see any symptoms in the other eye (if you only have it in one eye)?
- Will a change in my regular glasses help at all?
- What medical/surgical treatment might be appropriate for me?
- Should I watch for any particular symptoms and notify you if they occur?
- If my vision can't be corrected, can you refer me to a specialist in low vision?
- Where is the best place to call about vision rehabilitation?
- What can I do to protect or prolong my vision?
- Who can recommend a vitamin/mineral program for me that might be helpful?

Also review with the doctor what medications you are taking. Are any of them harmful to the eyes? Don't forget to discuss over-the-counter medicines. People with AMD should avoid as much as possible any drugs that thin the blood, including aspirin and nonsteroid anti-inflammatory painkillers like ibuprofen. Many older people take "baby" aspirin for their heart; most experts feel that the quantity is too small to harm the eyes.

If you're on blood-thinning medicines, talk to both your internist and your ophthalmologist about alternatives.

What You Need to Learn from Your Doctor

Keeping track of your condition will be easier if you make a habit of getting a report from your doctor after each visit. You want to know

- current diagnosis
- visual acuity measurement—the 20/20 to 20/? measurement. Your "best corrected visual acuity" is a measurement of your vision with your glasses or contacts on.
- a description of the appearance of the retina and the macula
- any procedures that were performed
- any recommended medications or treatments

You can request a report directly from the doctor or from one of the office staff. To make the process easier, create a form listing each of the items above. You or the doctor can fill it in during or right after the examination. Make blank copies and take a new one with you for each examination.

Date of Exam _____
Current Diagnosis _____
Visual Acuity Measurement _____
Appearance of the Retina and Macula? _____
_____
_____
Procedures Performed? _____
_____
Recommended Medications or Treatments _____
_____

This information will provide you with a history of the health of your eyes. After subsequent visits you'll have a better understanding of whether or not your condition is progressing. In addition, if you should consult other doctors about your situation, your documentation will provide them with the information they need to help you.

Seeking the Best Advice

Unless you get a clean bill of health on the fluorescein angiography and related tests, you may want to start investigating if low-vision specialists or vision-rehabilitation centers exist in your area. Though this may sound premature if your lifestyle is not yet compromised, there is good reason to seek out professionals who are dealing with all levels of macular degeneration every day. Those who see variations in the disease are best equipped to analyze your situation, even early on. In addition, there are different tests that are conducted by low-vision specialists, and these may be helpful both in identifying ways to maximize your sight and in charting the progress of your condition.

A full-service vision-rehabilitation center such as the Lighthouse has diagnostic experts, vision rehabilitation specialists, and doctors who can prescribe appropriate visual aids for you.

To locate a center or specialist near you, call the American Optometric Association, the American Academy of Ophthalmology, or the Lighthouse (see Resources section). (Lighthouse International answers more than ten thousand calls of this type per year.) Your local Lions Club may also have information on resources in your community. Or contact your state's Commission for the Blind. (Don't be put off by the name; name changes take time, and they offer services for people with all levels of visual impairment.)

Unfortunately, some of the vision-rehabilitation centers listed on national resource lists do not offer a full range of services. A good one will have

- an eye-care professional on staff who is trained to conduct low-vision evaluations
- access to a wide variety of low-vision devices ranging from special glasses to hand magnifiers to technological inventions that enhance vision, all of which can be exchanged until the correct match between patient and device is found
- vision-rehabilitation professionals, including:
  - low-vision instructors and low-vision therapists to provide training in the use of devices
  - rehabilitation teachers to recommend changes in your office or home and training in the skills of daily living
  - orientation and mobility specialists to help you move safely about in the home, the street, and outside facilities
- social workers or psychologists to provide counseling

Most important, a good low-vision evaluation is totally patient-oriented. Questions asked should range from your current health to your lifestyle and eating habits. All the questions are intended to help the specialist ascertain exactly what you're having difficulty seeing and under what lighting conditions you function best.

Here are some of the types of questions you ought to be prepared to answer:

- What do you do during the day?
- Of the tasks you need to accomplish, what can't you do now?
- What do you want to be able to do? Attend the theater? Use your computer? Golf?
- What can't you read that you would like to be able to read? Be specific. Read a novel? Read the morning newspaper? Read prices at the supermarket?
- When you are outdoors, is it more difficult to see under particular conditions or at particular times of day?

The more information you can give to the low-vision professional, the better he or she will be able to help you. Take with you all eyewear you use, including dark glasses. The specialist may want to adjust your prescription or recommend a different-colored tint for the dark glasses.

In addition to the testing a regular ophtalmologist or optometrist performs, several additional tests are run during the low-vision evaluation.

Identifying Your Scotoma

If deterioration has progressed to the point that you have a scotoma, or blind spot, your low-vision specialist can work with you to identify exactly where it is. Later in the book you will learn more about learning to "see around" your blind spot, but knowing where your scotoma is located is also important in tracking the progress of your disease.

Glare Sensitivity Testing

Glare—that blinding feeling we all get when we suddenly emerge from darkness into bright sunlight—can become a constant problem for some people. A glare effect that hinders seeing does not result from macular degeneration, but because you need to reclaim all the vision you can, it is important that glare be managed, sometimes with a change as simple as tinted glasses. To test for glare sensitivity, the eye-care professional may shine a brightness acuity tester or an ordinary penlight into your eyes while you read an eye chart.

Contrast Sensitivity

The brain is very sensitive to changes in contrast, as shown when driving at dusk or reading the faded print of a newspaper. When affected by a disease like AMD, the eye becomes less able to see objects unless the contrast is strong. A patient may perform well on an eye chart, where the lighting is good and the letters on the chart are offered in high contrast. Upon entering a restaurant, though, this same person may find reading the menu virtually impossible because of poor lighting and delicate cursive lettering.

Two clinical tests are run to check for contrast sensitivity, and they take only a few minutes. One chart is made of letters; the other has lines. The figures start out quite dark on one side of the chart and become progressively lighter. The doctor records how much of the chart a patient is able to see.

As specialists in the field learn more about AMD, more types of tests are being conducted. Some vision centers are now testing the density of the macular pigment (layer of cells in the macula), since studies indicate that the breakdown of the pigment in the eye may mark the beginning of further damage to the retina. If this is indeed an early warning sign of AMD, doctors hope that remedies can be devised that will help prevent any damage.

In other centers, specialists are studying the effects of diet on macular degeneration. Some professionals are also testing various nutrient levels, to document whether or not dietary changes can make a difference.

Coming to Terms with Your Diagnosis

Every week new patients arrive at the Lighthouse proclaiming that they were "dismissed" by their regular doctor with the words "There's nothing more I can do for you."

Today if anyone tells you that, you can tell them they are absolutely wrong—even if it's your own doctor. The field of low vision is advancing daily, and you'll find there are many ways to make the most of the sight you have. That's not to say, however, that you won't experience feelings of sadness and loss.

"I was an interior decorator, so when I began losing my vision, including my ability to distinguish colors, I was devastated," says one woman in her sixties. "I remember trying to arrange flowers, something I had always been so good at, and I just couldn't do it anymore.

"Since then I've had to retire, and it hasn't been easy coming to terms with what I've lost."

Notes Dr. Lisa Weiss, a psychologist in private practice in the New York area, "Inevitably, a person worries about what he or she has to give up as a result of the disease. Does the person need or want to continue to work? How will this affect responsibilities to the family? Who will drive the person with macular degeneration to the doctor if that person can no longer do it? And what about reading the morning news-paper? There's real concern, and if these things must be given up, then there is also loss."

"I felt suicidal when I was diagnosed," says eighty-two-year-old Mary. "All my friends were having their cataracts removed successfully, and the doctor tells me I'm losing my vision from something untreatable. Why couldn't anything be done to help me?"

"The fact that macular degeneration strikes people later in life when other losses may be occurring makes it additionally difficult to accept," notes Dr. Stanley Wainapel, clinical director of rehabilitation medicine at Montefiore Hospital, who himself has low vision. "As Shakespeare says, 'When sorrows come, they don't come as single spies, they come as battallions.' "

Preliminary results from a Lighthouse study on depression and vision loss reveals that the foremost qualities that keep people from long-lasting depression are (1) good relationships with family members or a strong circle of friends, and (2) the willingness to keep trying.

"Disability leads to depression, and depression simply leads to greater disability," notes Dr. Amy Horowitz, senior vice president for research and evaluation at the Lighthouse. "The woman with a strong group of friends who are in and out of each other's homes several times per week will know that her friends will help her," adds Dr. Weiss. "In contrast, the man or woman who lives alone and whose children live far away may rightly feel that this situation could be very isolating."

Seventy-nine-year-old Sarah, a successful representational painter, was diagnosed with AMD ten years ago, and she went through a serious depression when she finally had to give up her work: "I continued to paint for another three or four years after I was diagnosed. Then, on a painting expedition to

Scotland, I set up to paint the landscape in the manner I usually did, and though I could see the beautiful, lush panorama I planned to paint, I realized I couldn't bring in any of the detail. I closed up my paints, and didn't want to paint again.

"Friends suggested I continue painting with a more abstract style, but I refused. My work had always been very disciplined, and I had no interest in painting bigger or more abstractly.

"I joined a support group, but I remained depressed for almost a year, and finally consulted my doctor, who prescribed an antidepressant for me," she says.

"Since then I've felt better and have found other activities to pursue. I decided writing would be an interesting type of expression for me, so I took a course to learn how to use the computer, and I now attend a writers' workshop regularly. It has provided me with a new and rewarding means of self-expression.

"Today when I enter a room and see only silhouettes, I remember the times when I teetered between rage and tears, but today I have adjusted to it somewhat. I am first to admit that half a loaf—seeing some things—is better than none."

Fear of losing independence can also bring on depression. "Being willing to be dependent some of the time is very difficult for some adults," says Dr. Weiss. "All our lives we've struggled to make it on our own, and when our situation changes and we must ask for help, many people have a very difficult time of it."

Ironically, many people really want to be helpful, and your accepting their help is a way of helping them. Think of specific tasks that will make your load easier, and when you can, match your request to the person who would most enjoy it. Tell your friend who runs a restaurant that you can no longer find a certain brand of tea you enjoy, and could he keep an eye out for it for you? Ask your neighbor who loves music if she would mind driving the two of you to a concert; you'd love to buy the tickets. People who have always been very independent are often surprised by how much pleasure they can bring to others by being willing to ask for help. The act of asking brings warmth to your relationship and helps build community.

For eighty-two-year-old Mary, who was quoted earlier as being suicidal upon her initial diagnosis, two experiences helped her gain control over her life. "A rehabilitation person kept reassuring me that I wouldn't go blind, that I wouldn't lose all of my vision, and that helped," she says. "The other incident occurred late one winter when I was leaving New York City's Avery Fisher Hall after a concert. I found my way toward the street and was about to cross when I heard a woman ask me to help her cross the street. 'I can't help you,' I said. 'I don't see very well.'

" 'That's all right,' she said to me. 'I see well enough for both of us. I just don't walk very well.' She took hold of my elbow, and we crossed the street together arm-in-arm."

"People shouldn't resist getting help," notes Amy Horowitz. "Depression is a disease, and if the situation isn't looking any brighter, it's important to treat it. If your depression (or feelings of loss and sadness) continues, it is best to consult a psychiatrist, who will determine the nature of your depression and if appropriate prescribe antidepressant medication or psychotherapy or a combination of both. Your regular doctor should be able to refer you to a psychiatrist. Coping with your depression can make it easier to learn new strategies for dealing with AMD."

"I Must Be Crazy . . . "

Another upsetting and little discussed side effect of macular degeneration is hallucinations, a normal part of the disease.

"I used to see small figures when I got into bed at night," says Margaret. "Some were tall, some were short; all were beautifully dressed. They were never frightening. At first I thought it was from medication, but they didn't go away, and I became used to them.

"I never mentioned them to anyone because I was afraid people would think I was crazy," she continues. "Then one of my doctors asked if I ever saw anything, and that's when I learned other people have had similar experiences. Then I fell last winter, and they have gone away. They didn't bother me, but I don't miss them."

The phenomenon of seeing hallucinations is called Charles Bonnet syndrome, named after the fellow who first identified it in 1769, when his father kept reporting that he saw visions. The Wilmer Ophthalmological Institute reports that as many as 15 percent of mentally sound patients with advanced AMD experience visual hallucinations, so you are not alone if you've been "seeing things."

The cause of Charles Bonnet syndrome is thought to be sensory deprivation. Lack of visual stimulation to the brain may cause it to send out electrical impulses that create these visions. In general, the person having the hallucination is well aware that the things they are seeing aren't really there, and the reports are almost always of pleasant visions.

Unfortunately, people are so worried about what they are experiencing, fearing that it is the beginning of some type of mental illness, that they never bring up the topic with their doctor. If they did so, they could be quickly reassured that it is a normal side effect of macular degeneration, not a sign of mental illness.

Explaining AMD to Others

Part of the predicament of macular degeneration is that no one else understands your experience—you seem to be perfectly capable of seeing and cleaning up the spill on the floor, but you didn't recognize one of your good friends at the holiday party. It is confusing to you and very puzzling to those around you.

As Henry Grunwald explains in his book about his own experience with AMD, *Twilight: Losing Sight, Gaining Insight:* "Once when my son, Peter, came to see me, he was surprised that I did not notice that he had started to grow a beard. On the other hand, I was able to spot that one of his shoelaces had come undone. 'I'm never sure what you can see and cannot see,' he complained."

"The fact that I can't recognize people easily since I don't see their faces is what distresses me the most," says Mark, who has had an eye disease with the same type of deterioration as AMD. "People accuse me of being standoffish or aloof because I don't return their wave if they see me from a distance. I wish people knew that I'm not being unfriendly. I just don't see them."

Use the pictures of this street scene—or similar pictures found in some of the brochures being produced about AMD.

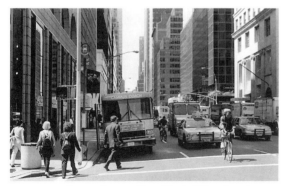 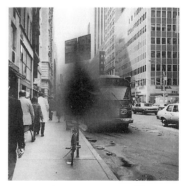

LEFT: An ordinary New York City street scene as seen by someone with healthy vision.   *Credit: Lighthouse International*

RIGHT: An ordinary New York City street scene as seen by someone with macular degeneration.   *Credit: Lighthouse International*

Show friends and family members how your vision is affected by macular degeneration. This will help them to begin to understand the difference between central vision and peripheral vision. You may soon find that they will help you hang a picture, but will no longer reach to help you every time you get out of a chair.

The National Eye Institute is currently devoting a large percentage of its budget to research on AMD and related diseases. The 1999 budget for NEI was $395 million, with an estimated $96 million spent on macular degenerative conditions in general and $25 million going specifically to AMD. As baby boomers enter the time of life when AMD commonly occurs, the NEI wants to find solutions as quickly as possible. According to Lighthouse International, by the time the last of our nation's baby boomers reach forty-five years of age in 2010, 20 million people will be visually impaired. Research in this field needs to come to prominence right now.

What follows is a rundown of what's going on in the field. Because progress is ongoing, I urge you to check the following Web sites every six months or so to find out if there is anything new to ask your doctor about:

http://www.amdalliance.com (sponsored by the AMD
    Alliance International)
http://www.lighthouse.org (for the Lighthouse Web site)

Treatment Options

Photodynamic Therapy (PDT)

Doctors are encouraged by this promising new treatment. Approved by the Food and Drug Administration in 2000, PDT is proving to be effective at stabilizing—not curing—vision in a certain percentage of people with wet AMD.

Unlike laser treatments that have been used for wet AMD over the last 25 years, PDT is revolutionary because the method permits the use of a cool laser, meaning that, unlike traditional laser treatments, PDT causes no damaging burns. In PDT, a patient is injected with a photosensitive dye that collects in the new, inefficient blood vessels. A nonthermal

4

Treatment Options

"So what can you do about this?" is the logical question patients ask eye-care professionals. Amazing advances in cataract surgery and all the advertising for refractive surgery (laser treatments that reduce the need for glasses) lead to the assumption that doctors must be able to "do something" about macular degeneration.

Unfortunately, there is no cure for age-related macular degeneration. One promising new treatment is helping a small percentage of those with wet macular degeneration (only 10 to 15 percent of those with AMD), but nothing at all can be currently done for the slower progressing dry form of the disease.

However, AMD is finally getting the attention it deserves. An impressive number of pharmaceutical companies (CIBA/ Novartis, Genentech, Miravant Medical Technologies Pharmacia Corp., Agouron Pfizer, Gilead Sciences, Alcon, EntreMed and Celgene among them) have dramatically increased research to investigate ways of slowing the progression of macular degeneration or decrease the degree of destruction of the central vision.

(low-energy) laser is then used to locate the light-sensitive dye and seal off the weaker, abnormal blood vessels.

The procedure takes about thirty minutes and is performed in an ophthalmologist's office. Although it needs to be repeated every few months, it can be done without injuring the retina.

In a clinical trial, 61.4 percent of those given Visudyne, the trademark name for the current light-sensitive PDT dye, and laser treatments found that their vision stabilized or improved, compared with 45.9 percent of patients in the control group.

Treatment is expected to cost approximately $1,200 a session, and most patients will require more than one course of therapy in a year. Because the injected drug is photosensitive, patients treated with it are warned to avoid exposure of skin or eyes to direct sunlight or bright indoor light for twenty-four hours after treatment.

Photodynamic therapy cannot repair existing damage, and unfortunately, the stabilization is not permanent. The other frustration is that at this writing, PDT can be used for only 20 to 30 percent of those with the wet form of AMD—primarily those who have had recent leakages, not people whose damage occurred long ago. Nevertheless, photodynamic therapy shows promise in an emerging field.

Eventually the PDT class of therapies may have several names, depending on the drug used to highlight the vessels. Currently, Visudyne (verteporfin), created by QLT Photo-Therapeutics and CIBA/Novartis, is the first to receive FDA approval. Several other companies are racing to get their treatment processes out in the marketplace.

Because no satisfactory treatment for AMD has been found, the FDA has granted priority review for several studies so that more options will become available. Among the other drugs that the FDA is currently investigating are the following.

PhotoPoint SnET2. Two drug companies—Miravant and Pharmacia/Upjohn—are developing this form of drug to use with photodynamic therapy. They hope that a single Photo-Point treatment will alter the course of AMD, making it less aggressive. The visual loss could be lessened, and the tissue may actually start to function again. Like Visudyne, Photo-Point is intended for use in wet AMD in which there has not been much irreversible loss.

Optrin. Like the other drugs, Optrin accumulates selectively in the diseased tissue, where it can be activated by light. A primary advantage of this drug is that it is water-soluble so it can be cleared from the bloodstream relatively quickly. This will help avoid the possible problems created by heightened photosensitivity.

Photocoagulation Laser Therapy

This is the traditional type of laser treatment that has been used for thirty years, helping to treat wet macular degeneration in a limited number of cases. It is most effective in patients with abnormal blood vessels growing away from the central retina, especially those who have clearly defined new-vessel membranes. Of those with wet AMD, only about 1 percent are good candidates.

In the treatment, a highly focused beam of light seals the leaking blood vessels that damage the macula. The procedure is usually done on an outpatient basis. After anesthetizing the eye using eyedrops, the doctor views the retina through a slit lamp similar to the one used for eye exams. Only minimal discomfort is felt as several small pulses of laser light are directed at the leaking vessels. Immediately after treatment, the patient may experience some increased blurring, but gradual improvement generally follows during the next few weeks. Between follow-up visits, the patient should check the Amsler grid daily to note any changes.

Although this procedure cannot cure macular degeneration, it can slow the rate of vision loss. Unfortunately, the surgery leaves a small, permanently dark "blind spot" at the point of laser contact.

Photocoagulation laser therapy has been described as a compromise treatment. A small portion of the retina is sacrificed in order to save the much larger area that would be damaged if vessels continued to grow. Success is achieved if the scar produced by the laser is smaller than the one that would have resulted if the eye was left untreated. Doctors have found that by using shorter laser pulses they can do less damage, but only about 7 percent of patients who undergo this treatment report successful results.

After the procedure, you will be permitted to leave the doctor's office, but arrange for someone to take you home. Your vision may be a little blurry, and your eyes may hurt a bit. The doctor will usually supply dark glasses, as your eyes will remain dilated for a while. However, you may want to take along your own dark glasses if you have an eyeglass prescription for distance vision.

The doctor will want to see you regularly following laser therapy and will have you undergo fluorescein angiography every few months to make sure that the blood vessels are not still leaking and that other blood vessels are not developing. If the vessels continue to leak, more laser surgery may be required.

If laser treatment is recommended to you, ask if photodynamic therapy is a better possibility. If your practitioner feels that the laser treatment is your best option, then don't delay.

Laser treatment is more successful if performed earlier in the progress of the disease.

Transpupillary Thermotherapy (TTT)

TTT is also being examined as a treatment for wet AMD. The process involves delivering heat to the retinal pigment epithelium (RPE) through the pupil by laser. It is similar to PDT, but the special light-sensitive dyes are not involved. A clinical trial is now underway.

Radiation Therapy

A number of research centers are investigating radiation therapy for wet macular degeneration. Because growing blood vessels are sensitive to radiation, researchers hope that delivering small amounts of radiation may halt or slow the leaking vessels. So far the results have been mixed. Critics are concerned about the possibility of long-term optic damage. However, the medical establishment is already using radiation therapy in the treatment of eye cancer—at four times the level necessary for AMD. At this point, no conclusive reports can be given.

Submacular Surgery

The goal of this retinal surgery is to remove the abnormal blood vessels that lie beneath the retina. To perform the operation, microsurgical instruments are used to remove the vitreous gel (called a vitrectomy) so that a small incision can be made in the retina in order to pull the abnormal vessels out of the eye. The vitreous gel is then replaced with a saline solution.

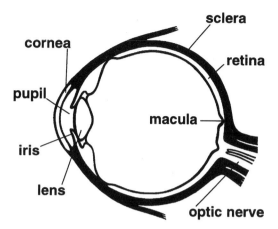

Credit: Lighthouse International

Submacular surgery trials sponsored by the NEI began in 1997; 1998 marked the beginning of the trials focusing on AMD. At this point, another two to four years of testing are needed, before there are meaningful outcomes. While the surgery has been quite successful when used for abnormalities in younger people, it has had mixed results in older people, who are the primary population group with AMD.

RPE Transplantation

The layer of cells called retinal pigment epithelium (RPE) is crucial to the light-gathering rods and cones. It is one of the first layers to be damaged when macular degeneration occurs, which then sets off the degenerative chain reaction. In a technique that has proven successful in animals, scientists are working on ways to transplant newer, healthy RPE cells to replace damaged cells, keeping alive the light-sensing rods and cones.

To perform an RPE transplant, the vitreous gel of the eye must be removed to gain access to the subretinal space. Then the patient's own functioning RPE cells, taken from the periphery of the retina, are injected under the retina. Next, the transplanted RPE cells need to arrange themselves to replace lost or diseased RPE.

This process is still highly experimental. The body may reject the transplanted cells, or the cells themselves may not adhere, and even if they do, it is not certain that they will do the new job assigned them.

Macular Translocation Surgery

This surgical technique involves moving the macula from the diseased portion of the retina to an area where the cells are healthier. After first removing the vitreous gel and cutting a flap in the retina, a surgeon then rotates and reattaches the macula to a healthier part of the subretinal tissue. It is still a very experimental process.

Laser Treatment of Drusen for Dry AMD

Treatments for dry AMD are sorely lacking, so this approach is promising. A laser is used to zap drusen (waste deposits that build up in unhealthy eyes). Researchers hope that by eliminating the potentially damaging drusen, the blood vessels in the eye can be kept healthy, and the progression of dry AMD into the more vision-threatening wet form can be slowed or halted.

The four-year results of clinical trials run by Iridex, a company that produces lasers for ophthalmological use, demonstrated that the accumulated drusen can be safely and significantly reduced or eliminated after only one treatment. Results showed that the drusen was eliminated in 78 percent of treated eyes versus 8 percent of eyes that received a placebo (mock) treatment. In addition, visual acuity was significantly better, with an improvement of two or more lines (on an eye chart) in 34 percent of selected treated eyes, compared with none in the control group.

Though this treatment must still go through additional trials before FDA approval, it is the first procedure that offers hope of some type of medical intervention for those with dry AMD.

Pharmacological Treatment

Many scientists believe that medications will play a major role in the treatment of macular degeneration in the future. The growth of unwanted weak new blood vessels, known as angiogenesis, is involved in over twenty eye diseases. Currently angiogenesis inhibitors are being used to halt the growth of cancerous tumors, and eye-care professionals are examining the use of this class of drugs to halt the growth of damaging new blood vessels.

A pharmaceutical known as AE-941 is currently undergoing clinical trials. Thalidomide, notorious for causing birth defects, and interferon are being tested to see if either of them can inhibit the proliferation of new blood vessels.

A natural protein in the human retina, called pigment epithelium-derived factor, has been shown to stop excessive blood vessel growth in rats. It will soon be tried for AMD.

Another promising drug is treatment with anti-VEGF (vascular endothelial growth factor), a genetically engineered antibody that destroys the cells that the body uses to make new blood vessels. Dr. David Guyer expresses hope about this drug in his introduction. Doctors are cautiously optimistic, because the drug seems to be particiularly effective for the eye.

Microcurrent Stimulation

MCS is a noninvasive experimental treatment adapted from FDA-approved therapies used to treat other eye disorders. In preliminary studies this treatment has improved both visual acuity and color perception. The process involves the periodic administration of pulses of small amounts of direct current at low voltages, delivered through electrodes in contact with the skin overlying key nerves around the eye. In early trials, patients were able to sustain improvements in vision over time by periodic self-administration of booster treatments.

Proton Therapy

Proton therapy is a radiation-like treatment (protons are the positively charged particles of an atom) that has been used in medicine for the last forty years. It has no side effects and is a standard treatment for ocular melanoma and other blood vessel malformations. The protons can be released very precisely and are aimed at a predetermined target site and depth. The therapy provides minimal damage to surrounding eye tissue and leaves no scarring.

In a clinical trial at Loma Linda University Medical Center, 89 percent of patients with the wet type of AMD demonstrated stabilization of their condition eighteen months after being treated with protons. Visual acuity improved or remained stable in 65 percent of patients.

Rheotherapy

Initial results of a pilot study of a controversial blood-filtering process, known as rheotherapy, were positive enough for the procedure to merit further examination. The procedure is based on the fact that certain patients with this type of AMD have elevated levels of some undesirable fats and heavy proteins. The pilot study was designed to see what would happen if the fats and heavy proteins were depleted from the blood. (For the patient, the procedure is similar to donating blood.) Pilot studies are too small to draw any definitive conclusions, so it will be a while before there is any solid data on this type of treatment.

With so much research under way, one or more of these therapies is bound to provide a breakthrough eventually.

If You're Eligible for Some Type of Treatment

If your doctor suggests that one of the treatments described in this chapter is appropriate for you, you'll want to fully understand the procedure. At your next doctor's visit be sure you get answers to the following questions as well as to any others that may concern you:

- What is the treatment process?
- What are the benefits of this treatment, and how successful is it?
- What are the risks and side effects?
- Who will conduct the surgery/treatment, and how much experience has this person had performing this procedure?
- Are there foods, drugs, or activities I should avoid before or after this treatment? (At the very least, your doctor will probably take you off all blood-thinning medication, including aspirin, prior to any treatment.)
- Are there any other treatments I should consider?

You must be careful of quackery, however. Bogus treatments are offered as "cures" for all types of ailments, and macular degeneration has its share of hoaxes.

In the next few years, legitimate new therapies not outlined in this book will be made available, and it's important that you carefully research anything new you hear about before you consider trying it. Talk to more than one medical professional before undergoing anything described to you. And remember, learning more about a treatment on a Web site doesn't mean anything when what you're researching is credibility—anyone can set up a Web site saying whatever they want to. You need to get recommendations from more than one doctor or other professional working in the field. Call the Lighthouse or the National Eye Institute (see Resources section) as another way to verify credentials. Remember, what they want to treat is your eyes—and they're important to you.

If you want to check out a treatment:

1. Ask your ophthalmologist, retinal specialist, or low-vision doctor whether he has read about it.
2. Ask the company or person suggesting the treatment to show you the professional journal that published the results of the treatment. The journal should be a reputable one in which all articles are reviewed by other scientists or doctors before they are published. A journal by a well-known medical organization will publish accurate reports, or check the front of the journal to see if there is an explanation of the article review process.
3. Are the only findings testimonials by individuals? If so, there is no fact-based proof that the treatment works.
4. Call the National Eye Institute to find out what they know about the treatment (see Resources section).

What You Should Know About Clinical Trials

Because people are eager for a "cure," many patients ask their doctors about participating in clinical studies of potential treatments for the disease. A clinical trial is a research study to test on actual people what seems promising in laboratory studies. Phase I of a clinical trial involves only twenty to eighty people, to evaluate safety and safe dosage of a drug or a treatment. Phase II clinical trials are increasingly larger studies undertaken to test the safety of the drug or equipment on selected patients. Phase III trials involve large numbers of patients who are divided into two groups, either receiving the experimental treatment or acting as controls. The control group receives a placebo (inactive treatment) instead of the therapy being tested. Phase IV studies are performed even after the drug or treatment has been approved by the Food and Drug Administration (FDA) and made available for public use. The studies continue in order to collect further information about the treatment and its effect on a broader group of participants and to study long-term effects.

Subjects generally have no control over the group to which they are assigned, and in masked studies (also called double-blind) neither the doctor nor the patient knows in which group the particular patient is enrolled. Location is a major factor for acceptance in a clinical trial. You may be a perfect candidate for a certain study, but if it is being conducted in another part of the country, your location may prohibit you from being selected for the study.

If you hear about a study that sounds interesting, you and your doctor should discuss whether or not participating is advised. You will have to sign a consent form that absolves the medical center of any responsibility.

First, you need a clear explanation of the rationale for the study. Then you'll want to ask:

- What does the trial consist of, and for how long does it continue?
- What risks are involved?
- What are the benefits? This answer may be twofold, direct benefit to you and long-term benefit to society.
- Do you have the right to leave the trial at any time? While you shouldn't enter a trial with thoughts of quitting, you also need to be given the right to leave if changes in your circumstances make participating in the trial difficult.

The government has a Web site that lists ongoing and forthcoming clinical trials: http://www.nei.nih.gov. The "Focused Search" function will help you locate people in your area who may be recruiting for ongoing trials. To locate trials not sponsored by the NEI, go to www.centerwatch.com.

If you're not comfortable searching the Internet, ask a friend or family member to help you, or visit the library.

As you can see, treatment options for macular degeneration are still in their infancy. You can expect to see improvements and, hopefully, breakthroughs in the future, but you don't have to wait. You can help your own cause right now. In the next two chapters, you'll find out the ways that people are helping themselves.

5

The Risk Factors of AMD and What You Can Do About Them

Specialists in eye care are looking to the past to find solutions for the future. It seems that investigating the factors that predispose people to get the disease may lead to some partial solutions. Observational evidence (information gathered by doctors observing patients, not through clinical studies) indicates that though the disease may not be curable, certain lifestyle changes may slow its progress.

Although there are no clear "causes" of macular degeneration, experts agree on a basic list of risk factors. While some of them are beyond your control, you can have a direct effect on the others. First, let's look at those we can't do anything about.

Risk Factors You Can't Control

Age

Simply growing older is the greatest risk factor of all. AMD affects about 14 percent of people fifty-five to sixty-four, 20 percent of those sixty-five to seventy-five; and up to 37 per-cent of those over age seventy-five. Yet while you can't control your age, you can work on being healthy and staying fit.

Gender

More women get macular degeneration, but this may be partially explained by the fact that women live longer.

Light Eye Color

AMD is more common in people with light-colored eyes. Because people with blue and light-colored eyes have less protective pigment in their eyes, they may experience greater damage from exposure to ultraviolet light.

Race

AMD is more common among Caucasians than other races, though researchers are beginning to find AMD in for-merly disease-free populations, most recently among Japa-nese and Brazilians. This increase gives rise to speculation that modern diet and environmental pollution may be strong contributing factors.

Genetics

If others in your family have macular degeneration, you have a greater risk of developing it. About 15 percent of those with AMD have a close relative with the disease. At this point, however, there is no proof that the disease progresses in the same way among various family members. If your mother was diagnosed as legally blind, you still have a chance to avoid the same fate.

However, because of this hereditary link, the American Academy of Ophthalmology (AAO) recommends that anyone who has a relative with AMD should have a retinal examination every two years.

Farsightedness

Because people who are farsighted seem to get AMD more frequently than those who are nearsighted, there is speculation that nearsighted people gain some protection from ultraviolet rays because they are more likely to be wearing glasses when outside. The protection lessens some of their UV exposure and may help decrease their risk for the disease. Contact lens wearers can achieve similar protection by asking for lenses with UV absorbers.

AMD in One Eye

If you have AMD in one eye, your chance of developing it in the other is higher. Studies are under way to see if anything can be done to prevent AMD from occurring in the good (high-risk) eye through using laser on the drusen or using laser to activate the RPE cells to clear the debris, but at this point there is no definitive answer.

Risk Factors You Can Control

Smoking

Smokers have a 50 percent greater risk of developing advanced AMD. Smoke restricts the blood flow throughout the body and interferes with the eye's ability to cleanse waste from the eye. Smokers also have lower levels of lutein, a carotenoid that is thought to be vital to the health of the eye. Research shows that the more you smoke, the greater your risk and the faster the progression of the disease.

High-Fat Diet and High Cholesterol

You have an increased chance of getting AMD if you have a high level of serum cholesterol. A high-fat, high-cholesterol diet can lead to fatty plaque deposits in the macular vessels, hampering blood flow and increasing the risk of AMD by 80 percent, according to a study conducted by the University of Wisconsin Medical School.

A heart-healthy diet is also an eye-healthy diet. Eat foods low in saturated fats and high in fruits and vegetables. (For more about diet see Chapter 6.)

Good Circulation

Good blood flow is vital to helping our bodies dispose of waste of all types, and this applies to the eye as well. To ensure that your eyes are getting an oxygen-rich supply of blood, you need to keep your heart pumping strongly. This is best accomplished through regular exercise. You can follow the guidelines put out by the American Heart Association and work up to exercising three to four times per week for thirty to sixty minutes. If you do not already exercise regularly, this is a good impetus to start. Check with your doctor about any program you plan to undertake.

Also, there is a strong link between high blood pressure and AMD, so have your blood pressure checked at regularly scheduled physical exams, and change your diet or medication according to your doctor's orders if you find that your blood pressure is high.

Exposure to the Sun

The invisible rays that cause your skin to burn will also damage your eyes. To protect your retina, buy sunglasses that offer as close to 100 percent UVA and UVB protection as possible. Don't take your sunglasses off even on overcast days. Just because the sun is hiding behind a cloud doesn't mean that your eyes are out of danger. Ultraviolet light passes through cloud cover and is just as dangerous as direct sunlight. Sunny or cloudy, the most dangerous times of day are from 10 A.M. to 3 P.M.

You may also want to consider sun-shield glasses that have side panels and a ridge at the top. These also help reduce glare. Decent-looking "wrap" glasses are available commercially. Recent Hollywood films have popularized a "wrap" style of dark glasses, meaning that you don't need to feel out of fashion.

The color of the lens does not affect the UV protection, though you should test whatever color or tint you select. Many find that amber-color glasses heighten contrast, which is important in helping people with AMD see better, particularly when outside. As you try on different glasses with various tints, make sure that none have a negative effect on your ability to tell colors. This is particularly important if you are still driving and need to be able to see traffic lights.

Your regular glasses can also be treated with ultraviolet protection, a clear coating that won't interfere with your sight.

In addition to wearing sunglasses, wear a wide-brimmed hat or sun visor. This will block about 50 percent of the UV radiation that would otherwise enter the eye around the glasses.

Macular degeneration is further complicated by cataracts, and protecting yourself from the sun may also slow the formation of cataracts. In 1988 a study was conducted on 838 fishermen who worked on Chesapeake Bay. The fishermen who did not wear glasses or a brimmed hat had three times as many cataracts as those who did, according to the American Academy of Ophthalmology.

Nutritional Deficiencies

Researchers are beginning to document how nutrition affects the course of the disease. A shortage of antioxidants, necessary substances that prevent damage to our bodies, increases the tendency for fatty deposits to stick to blood vessel walls, hampering circulation and the removal of waste products. This topic is explored in more detail in Chapter 6. Researchers are also beginning to think that certain nutrients are particularly helpful in protecting the retina. It is thought that lutein and zeaxanthin, available in dark green leafy vegetables, serve as "nature's sunglasses" and protect the retina from sun damage.

Self-Monitoring

In addition to making lifestyle changes, self-monitoring is a vital part of staying on top of your eye care. You can easily do so with the Amsler grid (see page 37). Your eye doctor will likely provide you with one, and brochures containing the grid are available from almost every major organization concerned with macular degeneration (see the Resources section).

Spotting a change in your vision when it occurs may mean being able to do something about it. Unfortunately, some people take the grid home, tape it on the refrigerator, and then take only a cursory look at it now and then. Others become too nervous to do the self-exam properly.

To be certain that you do self-monitoring regularly, at least twice a week, set a schedule for yourself. Note "grid" on your calendar for every Monday and Thursday, for example, or if you do the laundry on Tuesday and Friday, keep the grid near the washing machine and check your vision on the grid before starting your first tub of laundry.

Many experts recommend that the grid be taped on the refrigerator, so that it is convenient to check regularly, but Dr. Eleanor Faye, a well-known ophthalmologist and pioneer in the field of macular degeneration and low vision, warns that "People become overly accustomed to seeing the grid, and they think a quick look at it in the morning is all that needs to be done. Instead, the effective way to use the grid is to make an 'appointment' with yourself to seriously study it for a few moments. Holding it like reading material also permits you to check your vision more carefully than if you stand a distance from the refrigerator." Dr. Faye recommends the following:

1. With your glasses on, hold the card at the distance you would if you were reading.
2. Look at the card with both eyes. Note the dot and then look around the grid. Note irregularities. Are the lines straight? They should be. Do some appear wavy?
3. Cover one eye. Again, note the dot and then look around the grid, noting any irregularities.
4. Repeat the process with the other eye.

Dr. Faye also points out that while the Amsler grid is important, you can also "test" yourself more frequently by using objects you see every day. A wavy look to the venetian blinds in your office, or suddenly failing to see certain numbers on a wall calendar, are the types of vision changes that you should note. Any new irregularities should be reported to your doctor right away.

6

Carrots and Beyond: Helping Yourself Nutritionally

So many aspects of a disease like macular degeneration lie beyond our control. It's refreshing to find that there are positive steps we can take. For a moment let's review several of the central preventative points we've examined.

- When our eyes are exposed to too much light, damage to the cells of the macula can occur. Not just our skin needs to be protected from the sun; wearing protective eyewear is very important.
- A good circulatory system means a good heart, but it also makes for good eyes. Exercising ensures that the blood supply is getting up, in, and through your eyes.
- It's vital to quit smoking. Smokers have a high risk of AMD. At least seven studies have been conducted linking smoking with the development of macular degeneration.
- The food we eat also affects our overall well-being, including that of our eyes.

While the current studies are all observational (not clinically proven), people with a family history of AMD, or who have early signs of AMD, seem to be able to slow visual loss by eating nutritious meals, exercising, not smoking, and protecting their eyes from sunlight.

Since proof of nutritional benefits is not yet fully documented, the advice in this chapter comes with no guarantees. However, you'll learn about ongoing research and about nutritional changes the researchers recommend.

"Eat Your Vegetables!"

The folklore about the relationship between carrots and good eyesight may not be far off the mark. As it turns out, vegetables may help to prevent AMD.

As light enters the eye, it causes chemical reactions that activate oxygen and cause macular damage over the long term, a process known as oxidation, or "rusting" as we've termed it. "Free radicals"—molecules that are "waste" products of other working cells in our bodies—are what cause this unwanted oxidation, which, if unchecked, invades and injures healthy cells (in the eye as well as elsewhere in the body). We are exposed to free radicals through a range of environmental factors, from dietary fats and food additives to tobacco smoke and car exhaust. Even the simple act of breathing can create free radicals within the body. When a free radical invades a cell, it looks for a molecule to react with. If antioxidants—chemicals we get from vitamins and minerals—are present, they work to neutralize the free radicals before they can react with and harm other cells. If antioxidants are not present, the free radical will oxidize and damage other molecules, causing injury to the eye and elsewhere in the body.

Since they function as antioxidants, some experts feel that

consuming the following vitamins and minerals can help slow macular degeneration and other aging factors:

- vitamins C and E
- selenium (a mineral)
- carotenoids (family of compounds that includes beta carotene), especially those found in leafy green vegetables

The National Eye Institute has undertaken a study testing the effect of antioxidant vitamins and zinc on the progression of AMD as part of a study called AREDS (Age Related Eye Disease Study). Clinical trials are under way at eleven centers in the United States, involving 4,700 patients. The study's outcome is due in 2001.

Scientists have been researching other aspects of nutrition as well and have discovered that two carotenoids are particularly significant to eye health: lutein and zeaxanthin, important components in the macula pigment cells of healthy eyes. Unfortunately, they are not a part of the forthcoming NEI study, so government substantiation will have to wait.

The highest accumulation of lutein and zeaxanthin, carotenoid nutrients needed by the entire body, occurs in the eye. Because of the high concentration at the point of greatest visual acuity, scientists feel that lutein and zeaxanthin play an important role in eyesight. Researchers theorize that lutein and zeaxanthin protect the macula in two ways: by absorbing harmful blue light from the sun's rays and by acting as antioxidants that neutralize free radicals.

This theory is further supported by the fact that smokers, people with light blue eyes, and menopausal women, all of whom are at higher risk for AMD, have half as much natural lutein and zeaxanthin in the back of their eyes as the rest of the population.

This observation has encouraged researchers to theorize

that replacing lutein and zeaxanthin through dietary intake may provide protection for the macula. How does one get lutein and zeaxanthin? By eating vegetables, particularly dark leafy ones like spinach, kale, and collard greens. (Other lutein-rich foods are listed under the heading "What You Can Do" below.) Diets containing five to six servings of fresh vegetables per day can increase levels of lutein in the bloodstream by about 50 percent. In a preliminary study, people who consumed lutein from either spinach or supplements demonstrated some improvement of early vision loss caused by macular degeneration.

You may also soon be reading more about the benefit of eating tomatoes. New clinical research has found nutritional advantages in lycopene, an antioxidant found in tomatoes and tomato-based products.

Based on early studies showing that those who ate spinach three or four times a week experienced positive results within twelve weeks, Stuart Richer, O.D., Ph.D., chief of the optometry section at the VA Medical Center in North Chicago, has been conducting more in-depth studies on the effect that nutrition has on AMD. One is a study of ninety patients suffering from dry macular degeneration. Participants have been divided into three groups: one receives a placebo; the second receives a lutein supplement; the third receives lutein combined with other antioxidants.

Most studies must run for several years before conclusive results can be reached, but because lutein accumulates in the retina within a few weeks, Dr. Richer will release early results by mid-2001, and he is already collecting data from some patients who have reported positive changes in as few as six to eight weeks. For anyone with a diagnosis of AMD, the sooner conclusive information from this study can be released the better.

Some of Dr. Richer's early data conform with the European literature and agree with studies in the United States

demonstrating that people who eat little fruit and vegetables are at risk for AMD. A recent population-based cross-
sectional survey further substantiates this finding. AMD is lower
in self-sustained farming communities, where the population
primarily exists on the vegetables they grow, than elsewhere
in the industrial world.

What You Can Do

Dark green leafy vegetables, such as spinach, kale, turnip
and collard greens, are good sources of lutein and zeaxanthin. In addition to these foods, other sources include the
following: corn, kiwi, pumpkin, zuchini squash, yellow squash,
red grapes, green peas, cucumber (a dark horse since it's low
in other nutrients), butternut squash, green bell pepper, and
celery.

Other foods with beneficial carotenoids are carrots, can-
taloupe, sweet potatoes, and dried apricots. Tomato and tomato
products have only a little lutein and zeaxanthin, but they are
very high in lycopene, another carotenoid that may benefit
the eyes.

Surprisingly, egg yolks are also rich in lutein and zeaxanthin
(though only slightly more so than corn). However, since most
people need to watch their cholesterol levels, eating eggs for
lutein and zeaxanthin should be an occasional option, not a
regular one. An egg yolk has 215 milligrams of cholesterol out
of a recommended daily allowance of only 300. According to
the American Heart Association, people with healthy blood
cholesterol can eat as many as four eggs a week. However,
whenever possible get your carotenoids from a wide variety of
fruits and vegetables that have many additional nutritional
benefits, including fiber.

In general, consuming a diet that is rich in fruits and vegetables is the best way to get the nutrients you need. Here's a partial rundown of vitamins and minerals that are helpful to the eyes and what to eat to get them:

Vitamin A
  liver, egg yolks, fortified milk, dairy products, margarine, fish oil
Beta Carotene
  carrots, sweet potatoes, spinach and other dark green leafy vegetables, cantaloupes, apricots
Vitamin C
  citrus fruits, melons, berries, peppers, potatoes, cabbage, broccoli, tomatoes, some cereals
Vitamin D
  Vitamin D–fortified milk, egg yolks, eel, herring, salmon, liver
Vitamin E
  vegetable oil, nuts, wheat germ, whole grains, green leafy vegetables
Niacin
  meats, fish, liver, dried beans and peas, fortified grain products, nuts, potatoes
B6
  poultry, fish, whole grains, dried beans and peas, bananas, avocadoes
B12
  meats, dairy products, eggs, liver, fish
Folic acid
  leafy green vegetables, oranges, bananas, liver, dried beans and peas
Calcium
  dairy foods, some green leafy vegetables like broccoli and collards, tofu, calcium-fortified foods

Magnesium
    nuts, legumes, and some grains
Zinc
    meat, liver, eggs, seafood, and cereals
Selenium
    seafood, kidney, liver, other meats, some grains and seeds

Here are six helpful ways to change your diet:

1. Build meals around fruits and vegetables rather than around meat or carbohydrates (pasta, rice/potato).
2. The best fresh produce for your eyes is also the brightest. Pick the most colorful vegetables and fruits you can find—red, dark green, orange, or yellow. Strong evidence shows that these foods play a key role in keeping your eyes healthy.
3. Raw fruits and vegetables provide higher levels of nutrients than cooked ones, so keep washed carrots in the refrigerator and grab a bunch of grapes or an apple when you want a snack. The more fruits and vegetables you eat raw the better.
4. Dr. Richer advises adding four to seven servings each week of spinach, which makes an easy "add in." If you're having a salad, include some spinach leaves. If you're making a sandwich, add a spinach leaf instead of lettuce. Making soup? Toss in some spinach.
5. Invest in an antioxidant cookbook. You might want to try some new recipes.
6. Use fresh fruit as a snack—good for your eyes and good for your body.

So that you don't become confused, let's define what a serving is. A serving equals one cup of raw leafy vegetables, a half-cup of cooked or raw chopped vegetables, three-quarters of a cup of vegetable or fruit juice, one medium apple, banana, or orange, or a half cup of chopped, cooked, or canned fruit.

If you're attempting to consume a lot of spinach, kale, collard greens, and other fresh fruits and vegetables, try to eat organic in order to reduce your exposure to pesticides.

What About Supplements?

When it comes to supplements, you have two options.

You may seek out an expert who can make recommendations especially for you. A dietitian or a physician with a special interest in nutrition is a good choice. Some optometrists are beginning to specialize in nutrition and its effect on the eyes. Taken improperly, vitamins can conflict with each other, wiping out any good they do. In the worst case, vitamins taken in certain combinations or at certain levels can be toxic. If you're seriously interested in taking supplements, get professional advice.

Another option is to take a multivitamin or even a vitamin pill especially configured for the eyes and containing lutein; at least twenty such formulas are on the market. The "eye" vitamins sold at health food stores are more likely to have the right combinations of vitamins and herbs.

A Harvard Medical School study showed that people who ingested at least 8,700 IUs of beta carotene a day had 50 percent less risk of developing AMD. Many one-a-day multivitamin tablets have 10,000 IU of beta carotene, so even taking a simple multiple vitamin can help.

It's probably wise to avoid taking lutein as a special supplement above a dose of 6mg per day, because the side effects of lutein/zeaxanthin supplementation are still unknown. Doctors prefer that you maintain your dietary intake by eating plenty of fruits and vegetables.

Consult your physician before taking any form of supplement.

Herbal Supplements

If you read about antioxidants, you will come across herbal supplements like gingko biloba, grape seed extract, and bilberry. Each has strong antioxidant powers, and each functions in a different manner from the others.

Interestingly, we can attribute some of what we now know about antioxidants to what started out as "folk medicine." During World War II British pilots used to snack on bread covered with bilberry jam because they believed it helped their night vision. This folk remedy has since been proven scientifically. Research indicates that nutrients in bilberry can help nourish the light-sensing part of the retina, the retinal pigment epithelium. It uses these nutrients to accelerate the regeneration of the chemical rhodopsin, needed for night vision, which results in quicker adaptation to light fluctuations.

What About Zinc?

In the last few years, zinc has been the darling of doctors recommending ways to prevent macular degeneration. Zinc, one of the most common trace minerals in our body, is highly concentrated in the eye, particularly in the retina and tissues surrounding the macula. Zinc is necessary for the action of more than one hundred enzymes, including chemical reactions in the retina.

Studies have shown that some older people have low levels of zinc in their blood, either because of poor diet or poor absorption of zinc from food. Because zinc is important for the health of the macula, some doctors think that supplements of zinc in the diet may slow the progress of macular degeneration, but there is no agreement on this subject. Too much zinc may interfere with other trace minerals such as copper. Unfortunately, the authors of a recent study have concluded that oral zinc supplements should not be taken because of possible toxic effects and other complications. Again, any supplement you take should be prescribed by a professional so that the proper balance is maintained. Keep in mind, too, that some supplements on the market are of substandard quality, so buy from a reputable dealer.

This brings up a last point on this subject: What shouldn't you take? Review with your eye-care professional the regular medicines you take. It is preferable not to take blood-thinning medicines, but any change in what you're taking should be overseen by a professional.

Nonsteroid anti-inflammatory drugs such as ibuprofen may also not be a good idea. This type of medicine may cause retinal hemorrhages in eyes not yet harmed by AMD.

What Changes Should You Make?

As you consider making dietary changes, keep in mind that researchers do not agree on whether AMD responds to nutritional treatment and whether vitamin supplements or proper diet alone are the key to its prevention. That said, eating a healthful diet seems to be a simple enough change to make and one worth doing for your general health as well. Dr. Eleanor Faye reports that her patients who make lifestyle changes do show an improvement in the progress of their disease. That's a good recommendation to take.

As for the future, Dr. Frederick L. Ferris, Director of Biometry and Epidemiology and Chief of the Clinical Trials Branch, National Eye Institute, says that the use of vitamins does not promise a "cure" for macular degeneration. "Vitamins are going to have a small effect, like aspirin for cardiovascular disease, where you see a ten to twenty percent reduction in disease," says Ferris. "This might seem small from an individual perspective, but from a public health perspective, it makes a great difference. So reducing macular degeneration by ten percent for the individual would be a modest reduction in risk, but for the population, it would make a great deal of difference. The same thing would be true with cataracts. If you could slow the development of cataracts by ten years, I believe the projection is that it would be possible to cut the amount of cataract surgery in half."

By reducing our exposure to risk factors such as smoking, sunlight, diets rich in meats and saturated fats; by increasing our consumption of green leafy vegetables; and by getting lots of exercise, we can slow the progression of AMD and maybe even discourage its onset.

PART II

EXTRA VISION WHEN YOU NEED IT

7

Maximizing Sight: Simple Ways to See Better

An adjustment to her regular eyeglasses made a huge difference to Ruth. Emily found that a gooseneck lamp in her kitchen provided the additional illumination she needed to check recipes and identify spices. Ted found that by switching to books printed in a large-print format, he could continue to read with his regular glasses.

Some very simple changes can make a big difference in your ability to see. The alterations can be as basic as changing your bedside reading light, checking the prescription for your regular glasses, or wearing a sun visor or brimmed cap to cut glare when you're at the supermarket.

The place to start is learning more about the state of your vision. An appointment with a low-vision specialist or a vision-rehabilitation therapist can guide you in these activities, saving you time and some frustration.

Enhancing Vision: Finding Out How You See Best

If your diagnosis was made several years ago, or once you were already experiencing symptoms, you probably already know that you have a blind spot, or a spot where your vision is distorted, in one or both eyes. This is your scotoma, the spot where the damage to the central vision has been great enough to cause you to lose normal vision. Most people can describe where their blind spot is and its shape and size.

Because the need to see is so strong, most people are also quite good at working around this blind spot. If you find that you are sitting near and to the side of the television now, that's because you see the picture best that way. You've already learned to maximize your vision.

In a low-vision evaluation, your eye-care practitioner may work with you to better understand your scotoma. Under supervision, you may be asked to practice viewing objects with your peripheral vision. This process is a technique known as eccentric viewing, and it's a way of maximizing the use of your residual vision.

Practice Using Eccentric Vision

If you have nearly normal vision in one eye, you needn't attempt this exercise. Your "bad" eye is still giving you general peripheral information, and your "good" eye is focusing on the details.

But if you are losing vision in both eyes, practicing the use of eccentric vision at home will make you feel more comfortable in all that you do. Tape a picture from a magazine or a family photograph on your refrigerator, and stand about fifteen inches away. Experiment by moving your eyes in such a way that you find which direction allows you to focus best on the picture in front of you. Don't use any extreme movements of your head or neck, but if turning your head a bit one way or the other helps you bring the picture into focus more easily, feel free to do so.

- Look to the left but still try to see the picture.
- Look to the right, still trying to see the picture.
- Look up, still trying to focus on the picture.
- Look down, also trying to focus on the details of the picture.

You may need a few days of practice before your eyes find the position that lets you best see the picture. Once you have found this new way of seeing, practice it two or three times a day, perhaps just before or just after a meal. Ask family members or friends to provide you with new pictures to use so that you have practice focusing on delightful fresh images. You will find that your desire to see in the "outside world" will soon lead you to using this skill all the time.

Scanning

Scanning is another way to use your peripheral vision to focus on specific details. The process of scanning is something you have done every day of your life. Now you are going to do it systematically. (You may want advice from a professional on maximizing your scanning ability.)

If you have ever used a video camera to pan across a scene (to videotape a panorama as opposed to zooming in on a particular person or object), then you understand what is meant by scanning. When scanning, you may not see the most prominent object first, but you will eventually see the broad picture. With macular degeneration, the information gained through scanning will be more helpful if you scan in a predictable pattern.

Try sitting on a porch or a bench in a park where you have a wide view of things. As you look from left to right, do you see better if you look a little above or a little below the houses across the street? The answer will depend on the location of your scotoma.

Scanning is a key method for retrieving visual information of all types—when walking, when entering a room where a party is taking place, when arriving at a doctor's office. Once you're conscious of using it as a technique, you'll find processing the information you take in easier.

Double-Checking Your Eyeglasses

Once you've been diagnosed with macular degeneration, you'll want to be sure your regular glasses are offering you every benefit possible. Getting the prescription checked by an eye-care professional is the first step. Getting new glasses is the second one. Or perhaps you only need to have your old ones double-checked against the prescription. Mistakes do happen, and whether or not the lens is ground exactly to specification can make a big difference to someone with AMD.

You may want to consider an anti-reflective coating. Also ask about tinted glasses. Amber-tinted glasses (absorptive glasses) heighten contrast for people with AMD. These are generally worn for better vision outdoors, but in a paler hue, some people like wearing them indoors as well. Most also find that the amber tint helps greatly in making the transition from the brightness of outdoors to the darker lighting of indoors. Companies specializing in special lenses include Corning Medical Optics, NOIR Medical Optics, and Eschenbach Optik.

While you are getting your glasses checked, ask about getting new frames. There has been a revolution in both lenses and frames in recent years. Chances are excellent that you can be fitted with a lens that is lighter and thinner, and the frame itself can weigh next to nothing, making your glasses more comfortable.

People sometimes ask about progressive lenses (the invisible bi- and trifocals many people wear now), but most people with AMD find these increasingly difficult to wear because of the narrow area of sight within the lens for each part of the prescription. At some point you may find that you need several pairs of glasses—doctors sometimes recommend two, three, or even four pairs. One pair may be recommended for reading, one for the computer, one to watch television, and another tinted for wearing outdoors.

If your current eyeglasses still don't satisfy your needs, a low-vision specialist has many other options to offer you. Remember, even a 5 to 10 percent improvement in vision can make a big difference.

What You Need to Know About Light

If you're like most people with AMD, you need extra light in your life. On average, older people need about three times more light to see by than younger people do, and if you have macular degeneration you may want still more illumination.

Adding light to a room doesn't have to entail calling in an electrician. While additional ambient light can be helpful at times, lamps are actually more useful because closer light is stronger, and with the right lamp the light can be directed at exactly what you would like to see. While a gooseneck lamp next to your easy chair may not be in keeping with the rest of your living room decor, you'll find that you'll be able to see much better with it there.

Ambient light, or room light, helps you move safely around a room, but task lighting is required for close work. If you're reading, working at a hobby, paying bills, or playing cards, the most helpful light is one that can be aimed directly at what you are doing. Experiment with gooseneck, adjustable-arm, and clip-on lamps to see what works for you.

There are four basic variables in creating illumination:

1. *The source and the strength of the light.* A room bathed in natural sunlight provides the best light for seeing. With artificial lighting, the light needs to be matched to the purpose. For example, a ceiling light is not best suited for reading.

2. *Where you are in relation to the light.* In general, light from behind your shoulder is best, but you have to position yourself so that you don't cast a shadow. And if your vision is fading, then light focused directly on an object will be best.

3. *The positioning and angle of the light.* If you're doing close work—or as it becomes more difficult to see—you may find that the way to see best is to shine light directly onto what you want to see. The closer you place the light to the material and the more perpendicular the source to the material, the greater the increase in the amount of available light. Good lighting is generally achieved by placing the bulb about a foot away from the task or page. If the light is positioned badly, you may get glare. Experiment to find the best solution for you.

4. *The item being illuminated.* Shiny paper can cause a reflection. Dark yarn for knitting can be more difficult to work with than light-colored. Maybe what you're looking at is causing the problem.

Making adjustments in any one of these areas can make a big difference in how well you see. As you work to increase and improve your task lighting, also increase the general lighting in the room around you. Otherwise, the changeover from your task area to the room in general will give you the same "blinding" feeling as entering a darkened theater.

Selecting the Right Bulb

The right type of lightbulb is an individual matter; the choice depends on your vision as well as what you would like to see. To make a selection, visit a lighting store or a low-vision shop where a clerk will take time to show you the differences. Later on, you may find that the bulbs you like are available at the supermarket or a hardware store.

Take a book, some mail, or a medicine bottle with you so that you can run a more realistic test on what type of lighting works best for you. Here are the available choices.

Incandescent. This is the most common type of lightbulb. Most of the lights you have in your home are probably incandescent. Still, at the store you will want to see an example of incandescent lighting so that you'll have a basis for comparing the other types of lights.

These bulbs are inexpensive and easily available at all types of stores. In the proper wattage, they offer a comfortable ambient light for ceiling fixtures. Bear in mind, though, the light they give off has a yellow-ish hue that may not be ideal for some people with AMD. Incandescents also give off some heat, which may be a consideration if you're considering using the bulb in a lamp right beside you.

Fluorescent. Your memory of fluorescent lights may be of a flickering cool glow often used in schools and basements. Today new, greatly improved fluorescent bulbs are on the market; some are even designed so they can be used as a screw-in replacement for incandescent bulbs. Many people find that the new "warm" style of fluorescent causes less glare; others like these bulbs because colors remain true in their light. The bulbs also consume less electricity, radiate little heat, last much longer than incandescent bulbs, and cost less.

Unfortunately, fluorescent lights aren't right for everybody. People who have cataracts may find that fluorescents cause more glare, because the ultraviolet light in the bulb makes light scatter.

Halogen lights. These give off a wonderful light, similar to daylight, but the current version of these bulbs burns very hot. They are more expensive than other bulbs but use less electricity. Halogen desk lamps can provide excellent task lighting, but because the bulb burns hot, some people find them uncomfortable. Ceiling fixtures are beginning to be created so that they can take halogen bulbs, and some people have created excellent task lighting by adding a halogen "high hat" (a light canister that is mounted within the ceiling) above a desk or kitchen counter.

The tall torchère-style halogen lights are not recommended. They can tip over easily, and because they burn so hot, they present a very real fire hazard.

Chromalux bulbs. Like the halogen, the Chromalux bulb gives off an excellent white light, and it offers the benefit of being cool. Chromalux bulbs are available in regular sizes as well as mini-floodlight (most people prefer a 100-watt Chromalux or a mini-floodlight). Many find that Chromalux light enhances the contrast of print, making it look darker.

Finding the Proper Lamp

Once you've selected a type of bulb, you need to find the right type of lamp. You should test various styles of lamps. There are many types of utilitarian desk/table lamps on the market today.

Consider, for example, whether you need a gooseneck lamp you can aim directly at your work. Another consideration is finding lamps with reflectors inside. The reflector should enhance the illumination. You should always use a shaded lamp to reduce glare.

Once you choose the bulbs and lamps, make sure you match the wattage of the bulbs with what the lamps will take. High wattage in a lamp meant for a 60-watt bulb is a fire hazard. In new lamps look for labels in or near the socket that tell what the maximum wattage is. The notation isn't easy to read, so you may want to ask someone to provide you with the information. If you're using a lamp you already own, see if there is any information on the lamp. If not, the bulb you now use is probably the right wattage.

Glare Management

Glare can be a real problem for older people, but particularly those with AMD. There are several solutions.

A primary one is determining what time of day is particularly bad for you. If you still drive, you may need to avoid driving at that time, or certainly to avoid driving directly into the sun at that hour.

There are also special anti-glare sunglasses that come in a variety of tints. These glasses look like tinted safety glasses and can be worn alone or over a pair of corrective lenses. They cut out glare from the sides as well as from the top of the glasses. Work with your eye-care professional to select the tint that is right for you.

A hat or a visor can be very helpful in preventing glare. Some visors attach to your glasses; others incorporate polarized flip-up sunwear in the visor design. If you're bothered by the glare of the fluorescent lights in the supermarket, try wearing a sun visor or cap while shopping.

If you have one eye that is more bothered by glare than the other, some doctors suggest wearing an occluder (a patch) that fits over the lens of the susceptible eye. This will permit you to see out of one eye without glare bothering the other.

Make Your Household Objects User-Friendly

You may need to use specially designed optical equipment, such as a magnifying glass, a reading machine or a special computer program, to improve your ability to see, but before you consider these, you may want to attack the problem from the opposite direction. You can find products that are easier to see because they are bigger or because you can operate them by using peripheral vision.

For instance, is it difficult for you to see your watch? Look for one with a larger face. Companies also make watches with higher contrast.

Are you finding the TV remote and VCR programmer hard to use? Many mail-order catalogs now carry what they call a "universal remote," which features large keys.

In fact, there is a whole host of such products. Visit a specialty store or send for the catalogs featured in the Resources section. You can buy large-faced clocks, easy-to-read blood-pressure monitors, and magnifying mirrors. In addition, many objects—ranging from watches and calculators to bathroom scales—come now in designs that "talk," so you don't need to read them at all.

You can even do some talking yourself. Pick up a small tape recorder that is easy to use. These can be handy "memo pads" for keeping track of various projects during the day.

What about those electrical and telephone bills you so love paying? Not only can you get enlarged telephone dials, but most utility companies also print a large-type format for their bills. Call and see if yours does. (See Chapter 11 for additional suggestions.)

Finally, do you miss playing games with the grandchildren? Oversized games are now on the market. You are not alone. Once you start looking, you'll be surprised by how much there is to find.

How about the simple principle of dark on light? By heightening contrast, you can easily and effectively make objects more visible. By placing light objects on dark backgrounds and vice versa, you will almost always improve your ability to see them.

The specialty stores listed in the Resources section, plus many hardware and kitchen stores, sell a lightweight rubber matting that comes in many colors. Sold by the roll, the matting can be cut to size and placed under objects to add contrast. A dark mat under a light-colored telephone can become a permanent fixture, or a mat you keep in the kitchen can be brought out on an as-needed basis to provide contrast under cutting boards, plates, or anything else that you want to see better.

Reading Made Easier

Many people with AMD are able to continue to read, though eventually adaptive aids recommended by a professional may be necessary.

The next chapter outlines a host of low-vision devices for reading. First, though, you might want to try making these basic changes. When selecting reading material, look for

- high contrast
- adequate spacing between lines of text
- simple (roman typeface) fonts, rather than decorative fonts
- upper- and lowercase type (easier to read than in all caps)

- extra wide margins
- less glossy paper, to eliminate less glare

For some or all of your reading, you may be ready for large-print products. Today more items than ever are being created in large type. Refer to the Resources section and send for catalogs, or stop by your local library and inquire about what they have. In addition to books, *Time* magazine has just come out with a large-print edition. Other major magazines will likely follow.

The minimum size for large-print materials is size 14 type (compared to 10-point type, commonly used in regular printed material). Most large print is in 16- or 18-point type. You may also notice that you can see certain typefaces more readily than others. See which of these is more comfortable for you:

This is 14-point Times New Roman.

This is 16-point Arial.

This is 18-point Bookman.

This is 24-point Courier New.

So if you get letters or meeting reports from work or volunteer projects on computer, ask the sender to enlarge the type size.

You might also want to take a look at the new electronic books. After loading a handheld device with whatever titles you like, you can then adjust contrast and type size to make the electronic page easier to read. The idea of curling up with an electronic book may become more appealing when you see the benefits these devices can bring to someone with AMD.

Some people find that a device called a typoscope is helpful when reading. It looks like a piece of cardboard with a slot cut out of it, but what it does is isolate one line of type (or part of a line of type) at a time, to help cut down on any glare and make it easier for you to focus on what you're reading. Typoscopes are available from vision-rehabilitation centers.

Other "Reading" Options

You like having a clean house, but does this mean you have to clean it? This analogy might be applied to reading. While preserving your ability to read whatever you want to read is the goal of every low-vision practitioner, that doesn't mean you have to labor through every word yourself. What's important is the acquisition of language and information, not how you get it. Here are a few ideas to consider.

Books on tape are widely available in bookstores and are a highly popular way of "reading"—many drivers can tell you that. One man with AMD noted that he reads more now with books on tape than he did before his vision failed: "You can listen to audio books while you do other things," he says. "Now I can read while I shave and wash up in the morning, and when I traveled I used to put away my book toward the end of the flight because I got tired. With the audio books, I don't turn the cassette off until the seat belt light goes off and everyone is getting off the plane. I would prefer to be able to see better, but I've learned to turn certain adaptations in my favor."

Books and magazines are also available on cassette tape and recorded disk from the Library of Congress National Library

Services Talking Book Program. This is a free service to those who have been diagnosed as legally blind.

Some vision-rehabilitation centers offer programs in which volunteers are available to read to you. At Lighthouse International (see Resource section) appointment times can be booked. Some people not only book the hour but also their favorite volunteer. Over time, a friendship can develop. This program allows you to arrive with a stack of mail, the morning newspaper, or some reference material you need to examine, and the volunteer will help you go through everything.

You might not need to go so far. Sometimes friends can help out. One woman has a neighbor who enjoys recording books for her. Later they donate the tapes so that others can also enjoy them.

Last, the age of radio is not dead. Radio reading services exist in many cities. Broadcasters read the daily newspapers and local periodicals over special broadcast stations.

When it comes to optimizing what you can see, the glass is definitely half full. As a smart consumer, you have an entire world of possibilities open to you, once you consider things in a new way. Let's turn now specifically to low-vision devices, another world that will literally open your eyes.

8

Making the Best Use of Low-Vision Devices

The one sure way to get the most out of your remaining vision is to see a low-vision specialist (an optometrist or ophthalmologist specializing in the care of the partially sighted) for a low-vision evaluation and a prescription for proper low-vision devices. Even if you are undergoing medical treatment, such as the new photodynamic therapy (see Chapter 4), there are special devices to help you get back to work or take care of your everyday affairs.

Thanks in good measure to the video game industry, technology in this field is moving ahead by leaps and bounds. Let's investigate ways to help you see well enough to maintain (or return to) your everyday life.

In order to help you see better with macular degeneration, a doctor can use three techniques to enlarge what you see. These techniques are called *relative size magnification, relative distance magnification*, and *angular magnification*.

A book or magazine with large print, enlarged print on the computer, or phone numbers written in larger than usual print are examples of relative size magnification. Adding contrast by using bold writing in dark ink will make letters even more visible.

Relative distance magnification means bringing an object or something you're reading closer to the eye. When you bring the item closer, your eye (and your brain) projects a larger image or picture on the retina. Unfortunately, our eyes have difficulty focusing when something is brought too close, and that is where the low-vision device comes in. Strong reading glasses or a magnifier will permit you to focus on something as if it is closer to your face.

The third technique, angular magnification, is the stronger magnification used in binoculars that allow you to see a bird that is, say, 140 feet away. The bird will appear to be only 20 feet away with 7×35 binoculars. (The 7× is the magnification or strength of the binoculars and 35 is the size of the front lens in millimeters; this is what determines the amount of light that gets to the eye.) Angular magnification is also used for specialized telescopic devices that may be prescribed.

It is important that an eye-care practitioner make the appropriate determination as to what low-vision device is recommended. A shift in vision may have sent you to the store in search of a magnifier when in fact something more serious is occurring in your eye. **Make certain there is no new bleeding or any other medical condition that requires medical attention.**

As for low-vision aids, they range from the simple magnifying glass you buy at a drugstore to a high-tech binocular-like headpiece that uses miniature television cameras to show you the world. While you may luck into a handy magnifier at a stationery store that is perfect to use when you're checking prices at the grocery store, most of the devices should be recommended or prescribed by a low-vision doctor.

The person who works with you to select an appropriate

device should inquire about your goals, introduce you to the various devices, and help you select the ones that are helpful to you. The place should also offer training. Many centers will let you take a device home on a trial basis. If it doesn't work for you, you can return it. Call the Lighthouse International Information and Resource Service (see Resource section) for a low-vision rehabilitation or technology center near you.

Knowing how to use any of the devices is vital. If one of your friends says, "Oh, I tried one of those, they don't work," ask your friend this: "Were you trained to use it?" Chances are, your friend bought it "off the shelf" and, sadly, was never instructed on how to use it properly.

There are five basic categories of devices to consider. We will discuss the uses and advantages of each.

1. magnification
2. telescopic lenses
3. reading machines
4. computers with appropriate adjustments
5. adaptive equipment, such as a machine that reads to you

Magnification

Remember when you were a child and used a magnifying glass to see a leaf, a bug, or the hair on your brother's arm? You may remember that it took a few moments to find the right place to hold the magnifier when viewing the object and that good light always helped produce a clearer picture. When working with any of the following magnifying devices, those two principles will remain critical—proper viewing distance and good light.

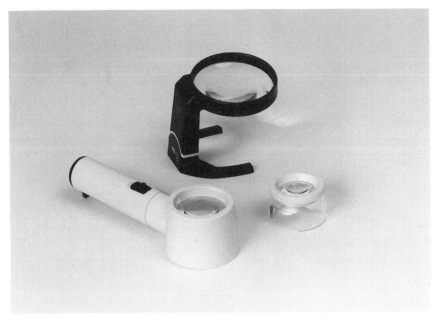

Some examples of stand magnifiers.   *Credit: Lighthouse International*

Hand and Stand Magnifiers

Hand magnifiers are detective-style magnifying glasses. Stand magnifiers rest on the reading material, and some have a self-contained light source. Both are good aids for short-term tasks.

Most people purchase these on their own, and their choices can be quite satisfactory, though your best purchases will be made when a professional helps select the right device for your use. Much stronger magnifiers are also available through low-vision specialists. Some dome-shaped magnifiers are specially designed to bring more light into the viewing field. Some come in a design that is long enough to show you a full line of text. Most of these devices are inexpensive, so it's worth trying a good number of them, and then once you've found a few that are helpful, place them around the house where you can

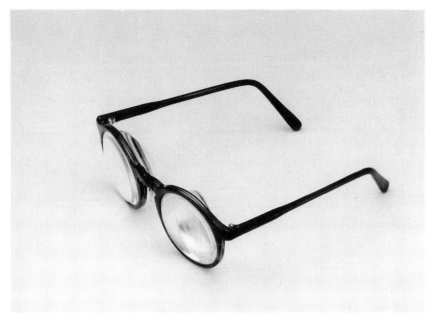

A pair of magnifying spectacles.   *Credit: Lighthouse International*

readily use them. If you're having difficulty making choices, talk to your low-vision specialist for recommendations.

Magnifying Spectacles (High-Plus Spectacles or Microscopic Lenses)

These are stronger than ordinary glasses and are designed for close work. You cannot wear them when you are moving around because you would become dizzy. Like the magnifying glass you used as a child, they do not allow you to see distances well.

These glasses can be made as "binocular" lenses for use with two eyes; doctors sometimes recommend "prism" glasses that permit both eyes to work together at a very close distance. The glasses look similar to normal glasses, but can be created to magnify objects three times.

If your eyes have difficulty working together at a close distance, sometimes a doctor will prescribe monocular lenses—that is, glasses that permit the good eye to work alone.

As vision decreases, the strength of the lens should increase. And as the strength of the lens increases, you must get closer to the page and the area you're trying to see (field of view). A general principle when using any type of magnifying device is that to be magnified effectively, the reading material needs to be brought closer to your face.

You will need to learn a little about optics, as well as some simple mathematics, to understand how the lenses prescribed by the low-vision doctor will work for you. We are all acquainted with the inch or the centimeter when measuring distances. But few people understand or have heard of the term "diopter." It's a term used to measure the strength of a lens. It is very important to understand the number of diopters prescribed, since this tells you how close you have to be from the print to see it clearly. The greater the number of diopters, the closer the working distance to the page. For example, a +2.50 diopter lens focuses at a distance of sixteen inches from the page, while a +5.00 diopter lens must be held eight inches from the page in order to see the print clearly. This measurement is called the focal distance of the lens.

The multiplication sign $\times$ may also appear on lenses and magnifiers. The $\times$ stands for magnification or the strength of the lens. A $2\times$ lens magnifies the print two times while a $4\times$ lens magnifies the print four times. One way of finding out the number of diopters in the lens is to multiply the number of the $\times$ power by four. For example, a $5\times$ lens prescribed by the doctor is twenty diopters ($4 \times 5 = 20$ diopters).

On the next page is a table that will easily enable you to determine the number of diopters prescribed by the eye doctor.

Magnification	Number of diopters	Working distance
1X	4	10" (25cm)
2X	8	5" (12.5cm)
3X	12	3.3" (8.3cm)
4X	16	2.5" (6.25cm)
5X	20	2.0" (5.0cm)
6X	24	1.6" (4.2cm)
7X	28	1.4" (3.6cm)
8X	32	1.25" (3.1cm)
10X	40	1.0" (2.5cm)

As you can see from the chart, the higher the magnification, the greater the number of diopters and the closer the working distance to the page.

How do you find where the lens is clearest for you?

1. Put on the new magnifying glasses the doctor has prescribed, and move your head down until your nose is almost touching the page.
2. Slowly move away from the page until the print is clearest. That is where the lens focuses.
3. Make sure that you are using appropriate lighting, especially if your doctor prescribes very strong lenses. (Ask him the strength of the lenses to get an idea of where they are supposed to focus.)
4. As with the use of anything new, training and practice are very important. If you have difficulty at first, keep trying, and don't hesitate to contact the prescribing professional to ask more questions. He will be able to help you make necessary adjustments.

You'll also find that keeping your head still and moving the reading material is a more comfortable way to read. Maintaining focus is easier if the material is what is a moving object and not your head. This is another part of the retraining process.

At first you may find it awkward to move what you are reading, but it becomes easier over time. You may have practiced hours on end to learn to play a musical instrument. The same is true here. You may have to practice to learn a new way of seeing.

Two advantages of magnifying eyewear is that people find it cosmetically acceptable, and your hands remain free for performing tasks. Such eyewear can also be used for prolonged reading.

Within a certain magnifying range, it is possible to continue to work with both eyes. However, at a certain point the strength may become such that using one eye is more effective than using both. The glasses can then be set up with one side darkened so you see through one eye alone.

Developing a system that works for you is a very individual pursuit, for you are the only one who can judge convenience. For example, because it would be difficult to move around the kitchen wearing magnifying spectacles, you might master a recipe in a two-step process: Read the recipe into a small tape recorder and then, while cooking, use the tape recorder to hear the recipe being read back to you.

Telescopes and Telescopic Lenses

A telescope? So now you have to look like a sea captain if you want to see something far away? Before you get carried away with an image of yourself standing on a street corner, peering through your eyeglass at a street sign with a parrot on your shoulder, rest assured that today's telescopes come in a variety of styles and sizes.

Telescopic systems magnify the apparent size of distant objects to make them appear to be closer than they really are. Some telescopes are indeed similar to those used by seafarers, but today's specialized telescopes are no bigger than the palm of your hand. You might slip one in a coat pocket, and

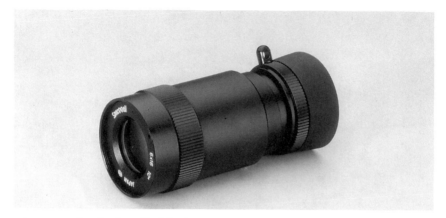

An example of a handheld telescope.   *Credit: Lighthouse International*

when you need to see a street sign, you simply pull it out and take a quick look before continuing on your way.

Prescriptive telescopic lenses are fit into the upper portion of the eyeglasses, a bit like wearing a strange sort of bifocal. They are used for distance magnification. Because of the nature of the telescopic lens, the lens itself protrudes from the glasses by a couple of inches, making it look a bit like you are wearing a miniature pair of binoculars.

Some styles, such as the pair worn by Victor Borge at the Kennedy Center Honors program in December 1999, are helpful for theater viewing. The bioptic telescope lens, with the telescope mounted in the upper part of the lens, is permitted in some states for use while driving, although careful training is required.

Reading Machines (Closed-Circuit Televisions)

CCTVs aren't actually televisions in the way we think of them. They are more like live television monitors. They look somewhat like the microfiche machines you might have used until recently at a library. The machine has a table-like surface

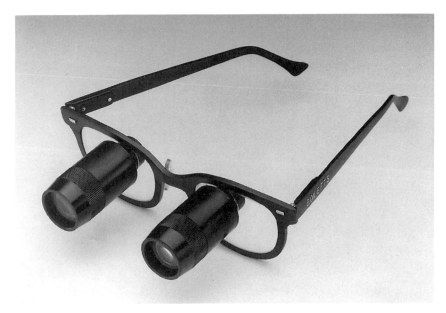

A pair of telescopic glasses.   *Credit: Lighthouse International*

on which you place whatever you want to read. People use CCTVs for reading books or the morning newspaper, viewing photographs of the grandchildren, or even filling out checks. You place the check on the flatbed of the CCTV, and the check can then be enlarged to the point where it can be filled out accurately.

Standard CCTVs consist of a camera and screen monitor (usually twelve to nineteen inches). Material is placed under the camera and is then magnified and displayed on the monitor. Print size, brightness, and contrast can be adjusted to meet individual needs. The image can be viewed either with black letters on a white screen or white letters on a black screen. Standard CCTVs are black-and-white, but color is also available.

The levels of magnification far exceed that of standard optical devices. You can get 25–40× magnification with a closed-circuit television. This compares with the 6–8× magnification

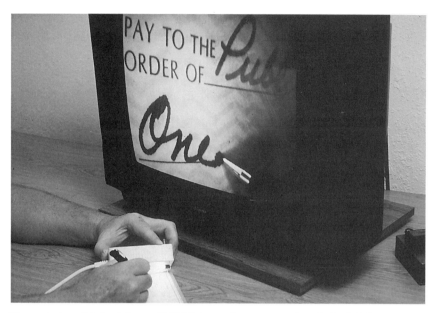

Closed-circuit televisions (CCTVs) can be tremendously helpful to people with macular degeneration. Here a CCTV makes check writing not only possible, but easy.   *Credit: Lighthouse International*

of a pair of high-powered reading glasses. In addition, the fact that lighting, contrast, and size can all be adjusted to suit your personal needs make the CCTV an ideal low-vision device.

Portable CCTVs are now increasingly available. Some use a small handheld camera that is passed over the text (such as cooking directions on a can or medicine dosage on a prescription bottle). The enlarged image then appears on a standard CCTV monitor, a small portable monitor, or on the screen of an ordinary television set or computer, depending on the model you select. This offers flexibility, plus the possibility of reduced cost, if you plan to use the device with your own television screen, for example.

One version of the CCTV combines elements of a scanning system with elements of a CCTV. Pages are scanned in at the rate of about ten seconds per page, and then the text is displayed in magnified form on a monitor. Text can be scrolled

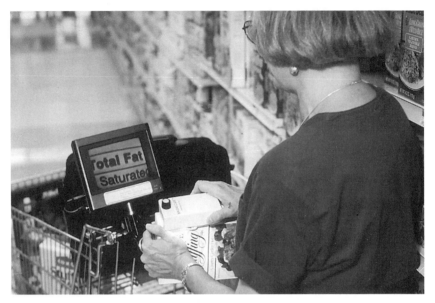

Here a portable closed-circuit television (CCTV) makes it possible to read the small print on a box in the grocery story. A handheld device "reads" the printed image, which is projected as a magnified image onto a portable screen.   *Credit: Lighthouse International*

continuously across the screen, making this a good choice for people who read a lot.

Certain CCTVs can be used with computers. Only one monitor is needed because the computer and the CCTV device can share the screen. If the user chooses to work with a split screen (showing both the computer program as well as the CCTV image), then she can read printed text and computer files at the same time.

For a standard black-and-white version, prices of CCTVs start at about $1,800. Portables vary in price depending on size and display capability but begin at about $900. The CCTV with scanning and scrolling costs about $2,900; this price does not include the cost of the monitor.

Video Headsets

One of the most technologically advanced low-vision devices to date is a video vision system, which you wear as headgear. Those of you who have been to video arcades may have seen virtual reality headsets; others might think back to their own childhoods and remember the Viewmaster. A video headset is like binoculars that stay on your face without you having to hold them.

This system offers the user great mobility. A portable CCTV permits you to scan whatever you want to see with a handheld camera, but to see the enhancement, you must be near a viewing screen. The advantage to the headset system is that the device is all-in-one. The headset contains the camera that captures what you are looking at—whether it's a crossword puzzle or your friend's face across the table—and projects the image on screens within the headset, right before your eyes. Because it enlarges and alters perception of objects, the device cannot be worn for walking around, but as the invention becomes more common, it will change the lives of those with macular degeneration.

The first of these devices was known as the LVES (Low Vision Enhancement System). The battery-powered set fit like a lightweight headset, much like the kind used in video arcades, and it had three tiny cameras mounted in it that reflected images in front of the eyes. You could adjust the set for both close-up and distance tasks, giving you flexibility. The image from the camera was displayed on small screens in front of the eyes, rather than through glass lenses. Both magnification and contrast could be controlled by the wearer.

The LVES, though, weighed an uncomfortable 2.5 pounds, and it was replaced by the V-Max, a 23-ounce system that provides continuous focus magnification up to 24×. It can be used for distance, intermediate, and close-up tasks. This version

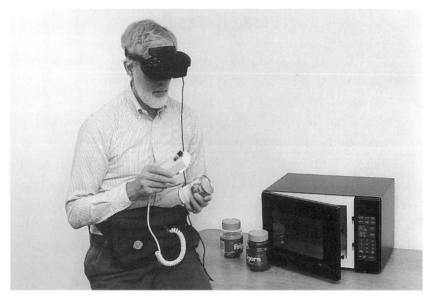

With a video headset a handheld device "reads" the label on the can and projects it onto screens inside the headgear, right in front of the wearer's eyes.   *Credit: Lighthouse International*

of the system also permits reversing the polarity of the print so that letters can appear white on a black background or black on a white background, whichever the viewer prefers.

The latest improvement to head-mounted systems is the Jordy. This system weighs only ten ounces, and is a full-color automatic focusing television system you can wear. It can magnify up to 24×. It can be used for seeing the faces of relatives or going to the theater, or it can be converted to a closed-circuit television for reading and writing. Another head-mounted system is NuVision.

With the portable units, you can aim the camera so that you can read around a pill bottle or the curve of a can. Each of these units is easy to use, although they do take a little getting used to.

Optical Character Recognition Machines

These personal reading machines look like small copying machines, but they actually have the ability to read to you anything that is typed—from a page printed in a magazine to a letter you receive in the mail.

The device itself has a glass screen on which print to be read is placed. The information is then scanned, and within a few seconds the machine reads the printed page, using a synthesized voice. It can read almost any book, newspaper, or other typewritten material, but it cannot read personal handwriting.

OCRs can also be connected to personal computers so that reading material can be converted into large-print or computer-accessible files. Test the OCR with the documents for which you plan to use it. They are easy to use but expensive. Prices start at about $4,000. Those that operate with your computer begin at about $1,500.

Computers

Many hardware and software devices can be added to your personal computer to make everything from a spreadsheet or word processing document to the Internet accessible to people with AMD. Microsoft has worked hard to achieve accessibility for those with vision impairment.

However, long before you start adding new software to your computer, there are some basic adjustments you can make with the programs you currently use. Start with the font size. If you can increase the font size to the point where you can read what's on the screen, you probably don't need to outfit your computer in any other way. And if increasing the font size doesn't make the type as clear as you would like it, try making the text bold. The increased contrast can make a big difference. Most computer systems are designed so that a simple adjustment can change also the contrast, creating white type on a black screen instead of black type on a white screen.

Also, if you add only one piece of equipment, consider adding a larger monitor. A bigger screen permits greater meaningful magnification. The larger the monitor, the more you will be able to magnify and still see a full line of type. At some point, even with a large monitor, the magnification may get to a size that you cannot see a full line; there is no doubt that this is inconvenient, but at this writing, there is no solution.

What about those people who can't see the cursor easily? Long before computer users became accustomed to the mouse, which requires careful placing of the cursor on screen, computers were designed to operate using keystrokes. Consult a friend or sign up for a computer class where you can relearn the key strokes for various commands. (See below for other options including enlarging your cursor.)

In general, you should consult a vision rehabilitation agency to learn more about how best to adapt your computer. Here are several topics you might want to raise:

Large print or screen magnification devices. These can be either hardware or software additions, and they permit an enlargement of the text beyond what regular adjusting of the font will do. Customized larger cursors are also available from various sites. Type in the search word "cursor" on the Internet to find helpful sites. Or, for more information about large-print programs as well as information on large cursors, visit the following Web site: http://www.magnifiers.org.

Text-to-speech and speech-to-text software. A hardware or software synthesizer "reads" the screen via its computer-generated voice. It also "navigates" the screen—that is, it announces cursor location and the highlighted item and monitors other computer functions.

For this technology you will need to add a synthetic voice drive. You will likely need both a synthesizer (hardware) and software that runs the speech drive. Plus, the hard- and software must be compatible. If you have Windows 95, 98, or 2000 or Windows NT, the synthesizer can make use of the sound system that is already part of the PC, thus saving money.

First created for the visually impaired, these programs are becoming popular with the "carpal tunnel set," that is those who have developed wrist injuries from too much keyboarding. That's good news, because the greater the need, the lower the price and the more work that goes into developing the technology. In addition, this program permits consumers to retrieve their e-mail by phone, to program household devices, and to speak to business colleagues around the world in various languages. In future, a customer will be able to dictate a letter over the phone and have it sent as an e-mail text message.

Internet conversion programs. Navigating the Internet has been made easier because of new programs that translate what's on the Web page into voice descriptions. Screen-reading software can vary from $450 to $1,400, depending on the quality of the voice and other issues. Be sure hardware and software you add is compatible with the rest of your system.

Selecting the Devices That Are Right for You

Because success in using the device is so important, when you call any vision-rehabilitation center, be sure to ask the following:

- Is someone available to help explain my best options?
- Is training included as part of the service?
  If the person assures you that something will be "easy to use and you won't need training," see if other centers

exist in your area. The devices are not necessarily complicated to use, but fully understanding their use can make your life easier. Think of how frustrated we all are when our computer starts acting up. You don't want that feeling with your low-vision device.

- May I take the device home on a trial basis?
  A reputable center will be eager for you to succeed with the device. You should be encouraged to try devices on a trial basis. If it isn't working for you, maybe adjustments can be made or perhaps another device will be more helpful to you.

Keep in mind that a device that works for others may not work for you. Consult with your eye-care specialist before purchasing any equipment. She may have comments about your vision and whether a device will help your specific problem.

Cost is another factor. Some hand magnifiers cost only a few dollars, but electronic devices can cost several thousand. At this writing, Medicare does not cover the services of vision-rehabilitation therapists or the cost of low-vision devices. The National Vision Rehabilitation Cooperative is spearheading a major campaign to rectify this oversight. More information about what you can do to support this campaign is provided in the Resource section.

To summarize: Specialized training is vital to success, yet many places aren't prepared to offer it since it is not covered by Medicare. First, the low-vision specialist needs to evaluate your goals and decide what will work best for you. Then the two of you must work together to make certain you're using the device correctly. After that, there's work left for you to do on your own—not every device will feel "natural," but if you continue to practice using it, it will become easier.

Thinking Through Your Needs

Chapter 3 discusses finding a medical professional who specializes in low vision. He may also be the one who helps you evaluate low-vision devices. This person—or the vision-rehabilitation therapist assigned to help you—should be very interested in what you want to see. For the next few days, make notes about what you're having difficulty doing.

- Are you still driving, and if so, do you have any particular worries about it?
- Do you have any difficulty getting around by foot? Crossing streets? Seeing bus signs? Seeing street signs?
- Around the house:
  - Do you have difficulty with routine chores? With personal grooming?
  - Can you see the television well enough (if you watch TV)?
- Do you still work? Are there tasks you perform at work that are now more difficult?
- Is there close-up work you'd like to be able to see better?
  - Newspaper?
  - Magazines?
  - Recipes, directions?
  - Sewing?
  - Books?
  - Check writing?
  - Using the telephone? Reading the phone book?
  - Reading the mail or paying bills?
- Can you still participate in your hobbies to your satisfaction?

Based on this analysis, set specific goals about what you want to accomplish. What are your priorities at this moment?

Once you've mastered those, you can formulate a new set of goals.

When you meet with the low-vision specialist, actively participate in the discussion. For these devices to serve you best, you need to make your likes and dislikes known. If something doesn't feel comfortable, say so. Perhaps an adjustment can be made, or maybe you can try another option—just keep pushing until you're satisfied. That's what a good center is there for.

Practicing with Your New Device

1. Make sure that you know how strong the lenses are that were prescribed by the eye doctor.
2. Check the diopter chart (page 109) so that you know where to hold the print.
3. Use a good adjustable light. Place the light so that it is about eight to twelve inches from the page and make sure there is no glare.
4. Understand that reading becomes progressively more difficult as the number of diopters increases. The reason for this is that as the strength increases, fewer words are seen at one time.
5. Try to move the print, not your eyes.
6. Try to keep the lens parallel to the page. That is, do not tilt the lens.
7. Practice and practice some more.
8. Start with headlines in the newspaper or with the large print in some of your favorite magazines because the print is blacker. That is, the print has better contrast. This exercise will help you learn the new way of seeing with your lenses.
9. Another exercise is to circle letters in order of the alphabet. Start by circling the first large A you come across, followed by a B and C and so forth.

10. Work in short periods of time if you get tired. It is like exercising with muscles that you have never used. Build up your endurance by working in short sessions and gradually expanding the time.
11. Work to smaller and smaller print sizes.
12. Again, check to see if you are working at the correct distance. See if the lighting is correct.
13. Use a cutout guide known as a typoscope, available from the low-vision specialist, to help you keep your place.
14. Bring a list of questions to your doctor at the next visit. You may want help in pursuing other hobbies or interests.

Here is an important reminder. The use of these devices takes practice. The earlier macular degeneration is diagnosed, the more gradual will be your adaptation to a device. For example, if the disease is not advanced, your magnifying spectacles will probably begin at a lower power, meaning that instead of holding the newspaper within two inches of your face—as is necessary at some of the higher magnifying strengths— you can start with it eight to ten inches away. If your eyes should worsen, then stronger glasses and closer distance will not be such a hard adjustment to make. Your eye-care professional should also work with you on the basics, such as achieving a comfortable posture while holding something closer to your face.

Remember, too, that learning anything new takes time. Certainly in the beginning the tasks you are doing will take longer, and you may find that you can't increase your speed much more, even with practice. But consider the attitude of the seventy-nine-year-old woman with 20/400 vision in her good eye. After working very hard to learn to use her magnifying spectacles well enough to read the newspaper, she addressed the "extra time" issue: "It takes longer for me to read, so now I have two cups of coffee instead of just one."

"I Want to See Better but Look Normal"

To some extent that dream can be realized. Good glasses and magnifying glasses can be very helpful even as AMD progresses. But at some point you may have to address the fact that in order to see, you'll need to wear a headset or use very thick magnifying glasses.

If you do get to the point where the eyewear or device becomes cumbersome, keep in mind that these items aren't worn full-time, and they aren't as noticeable as you think. Only a knowledgeable television viewer would have realized that Victor Borge was wearing telescopic glasses to see the stage at the 1999 Kennedy Center Honors program. As these devices become more and more available, seeing people— including famous people—wearing them will become an increasingly common experience.

Paying for Low-Vision Devices

If you can't afford the device that is right for you, check with your state or private vision-rehabilitation agency, state or local advocacy group, independent living center, or Lions Clubs International. They may have resources to help you, or have access to secondhand machines. You can also contact Lighthouse International (see Resources section) to request a free copy of "Grants-in-Aid," a resource guide that lists all the foundations and other organizations to which you can apply for financial assistance.

While a major campaign is underway to get low-vision devices covered under Medicare, only a few people who have purchased them have been able to receive any of this kind of funding. If you want to help change this situation, here's what you can do:

Eye-care professionals are increasingly prescribing electronic magnification systems such as CCTVs as prosthetic devices to replace the dysfunctional portion of the eye for people who are visually impaired. Medicare reimburses a range of assistive devices, referred to as "durable medical equipment," including prosthetic limbs, walkers, home glucose monitors, and much more. At this writing, however, optical devices and equipment for vision impairment are not reimbursed.

As more people pursue Medicare coverage under durable medical equipment, the current rules may eventually be changed. Increasingly, people who go through the following process are meeting with success. Your best opportunity is to follow the advice offered by Lighthouse International:

First, obtain and file the patient request for medical payment, HCFA FORM 1490, available at any Social Security or Medicare office.

Then ask your doctor (optometrist or ophthalmologist) to provide you with a prescription for the CCTV or other device, stating that it serves as a prosthesis for the dysfunctional portion of your eye and is required to assist you in reading medication information, prescriptions, and other tasks related to managing your medical needs.

Send in the request for payment form, the prescription (make sure the prescription date is before the date of purchase of your CCTV), the invoice, and your canceled check or proof of other form of payment. Send it all certified mail, return receipt requested.

You may have to follow up on the status of your claim, and eventually, it will almost certainly be denied. Ask at that point that they put the denial in writing. You won't be able to continue the appeals process if you don't have a written letter from the agency.

Once you've received a written denial, request a reconsideration and send along the same materials. You can add new information about your eye condition, and include a strongly worded letter from your eye-care professional.

When your reconsideration request is denied, ask for a hearing. It will be granted. Bring a family member, your doctor, or a close friend to help you plead your case. In almost all cases you will be denied once again, but according to advocates, you will have helped the cause.

With this next rejection, you can request a hearing before an administrative law judge. This is where advocates are beginning to see a change. At this stage, be sure to contact Lighthouse International (see Resources section) for updated information that may help your case.

Share this information and procedure with other people you know who are experiencing the same frustration. The more pressure we put on the government to treat a visual impairment the way it would any other type of disability, the sooner will come long-term change.

The Future of Vision Devices

The technology to aid people with low vision is moving ahead by leaps and bounds. We are entering the age of smart stuff—smart machines, smart spaces, smart materials. Scott Adams, the creator of the Dilbert cartoons, has been quoted as saying, "Pretty soon our clothes will be smarter than us."

This development can help all who are in any way visually impaired. For instance, navigational technologies are getting exponentially smaller, cheaper, and more powerful. The prototype wearable computers are now large, expensive, and not powerful enough to fulfill our needs. However, wearable computers or wearable appliances (head-, wrist-, or waist-mounted) are becoming less noticeable (blending with natural clothing), cheap enough so that consumers can buy them in stores, and powerful enough that many needs are addressed, maybe even without a professional to teach you how to use it.

Orientation and mobility specialists will be glad when rooms, desktops, the inside of cars, sidewalks, intersections, hallways—all become smart. Wearable computers will then interface, interrelate, and communicate with smart spaces. For example, your clothing might be embedded with computer chips so that your shirt could communicate with computer signals at intersections to tell you where you are.

Wearable computers will connect us to other people via telephone, pager, or e-mail access so that we'll only be out of touch if we want to be. Another useful idea is vests or belts that vibrate to indicate a clear path for the deaf or blind user.

Devices may one day exist that enable face recognition, and analytical software for wearable computers may soon have sensory enhancement capabilities, like digital video magnification, audio amplification, night vision, and ultraviolet and/or infrared vision.

The fact that many of these devices are being made for the general population is wonderful because this will lead to a faster drop in prices.

One day a machine may even be able to "run" the eye. Under exploration is a retinal chip that might eventually be implanted in the eye to mimic basic photoreceptor cell function. This might help people continue to get around even when they've been diagnosed as legally blind. Two forms of research are under way. One involves placing a retina implant chip over the photoreceptors at the back of the eye (subretinal implant). The other puts a retinal chip over the ganglion cell layer of the retina (the ganglia are the cells that carry signals from the photoreceptors to the optic nerve). Others are working on a totally artificial retina.

Don't give up hope. Keep eating a balanced diet (including lots of green leafy vegetables), exercising, and protecting your eyes from the sun—and stay on top of new developments.

PART III

PRACTICAL ADVICE FOR LIVING WELL

9

Basic Principles

Living well and—most important to most people—living independently with low vision means setting priorities and
creating strategies for accomplishing those priorities. You will
have a greater feeling of control over your life, and more time
to do what you want, if you begin by getting organized.

If you have macular degeneration, your days of performing
surgery, operating dangerous equipment, and piloting a plane
are ending. You may have other tasks that you really enjoy and
are sorry to have to give up. Other activities, from reading the
mail to balancing your checkbook, may simply take more
time. For that reason, it is more important than ever to set
priorities. If you never liked filling out your tax forms, this
may be a good time to ask someone to help you—or to turn
the task over to an outside accountant. Why go through the
struggle if you hated it anyway?

But if you want to keep playing golf, or even if you want to
learn something totally new—like writing a novel or baking
your first from-scratch cake—there's absolutely no reason why

you can't pursue those goals. Within reason, you can find experts out there who can help you do almost anything.

The information that follows in this chapter and Chapters 10 and 11 is the type of information that can be learned from vision-rehabilitation therapists. Nancy Paskin, Director of Rehabilitation Teaching at Lighthouse International, and her staff were instrumental in helping prepare this advice; many of the methods are also described in the Lighthouse International booklet "Whatever Works."

Though the guidance here is a good start or a great refresher, you will find these methods easier to learn and implement if you can be taught them firsthand. Vision-rehabilitation therapists specialize in many aspects of helping people adapt to reduced vision, and a professional can be instrumental in helping you learn independent living skills. To find someone in your area, ask your optometrist or ophthalmologist if there is a full-service rehabilitation agency in your area, or contact your state's Commission on the Blind (remember that name changes take time) or Commission on the Aging. Lighthouse International can also refer you to services in your area (800-829-0500). From cooking and medication to stair climbing and street navigation, your safety is paramount, so it's important to look for professional guidance.

Organizational Basics

Organization is key to functioning well in life no matter who you are or what your circumstances, but especially so with macular degeneration. The person who is organized will be able to find her orchestra tickets, put her hands on the recipe she needs, and keep track of everything from audio book rentals to medication bottles.

Your first step is to remember that the only things you need to organize are those things that are important to you. You need to be able to run your household, work (if you still do), pay your bills, keep track of appointments, fix meals, and get in and out of the house efficiently. You may have a hobby or an activity that should be added to this list. Don't bother with areas that don't affect you. Although cleaning out the basement might be good to do "one day," it needn't be a current priority.

Even if you are already an organized person, you may still want to skim through this section to see if the chapter suggests changes that will make your life easier.

Weed Out Your Living Areas

Most of us intend to throw out unnecessary items on a regular basis, but it's frequently a good intention that goes astray. Make it a priority now—again primarily in the areas where the clutter most affects you. Less clutter is guaranteed to make your life easier.

Set a schedule. Perhaps every Sunday afternoon you can attack one area of clutter that's bothering you. Write the job on your calendar so that the date is as ironclad as any appointment.

Set achievable goals. Your goal can be as small as cleaning out the kitchen utensil drawer, e.g., saving the bottle opener but tossing the tea infuser you never use. Or your goal may be more ambitious, such as sorting through and reevaluating what is stored in the linen closet.

This appointment with yourself might take five minutes or it might take two hours, depending on what you have chosen to reorganize.

Work systematically. If you want to straighten up the kitchen, make a list of the different cabinets, treat them as separate to-do items, and check them off as you complete each one.

Don't throw out anything you love. If you care about something, keep it! If it's a beautiful plate, you may want to start using it more often, or even display it. If it's a keepsake, you may want to think of a way to store it so that you and others can enjoy it more often. For the items you can't bear to part with but aren't sure why, establish a box for "On Hold" items to store in your basement or back closet. Two years from now you may sort through the box and say, "Now, why did I hold on to that old thing?"

Ask for help. A son, a daughter, a grandchild, or a good friend might be willing to help you sort through, weed out, and organize closets, cabinets, and jewelry boxes. For high-powered help, there are professional organizers who will come to your home and help you straighten out anything from your decades-old files to your computer system. Check the Yellow Pages under Professional Organizers, or call the National Association of Professional Organizers for a referral to someone in your area.

A Place for Everything

"A place for everything and everything in its place." Mothers have said this for years. This is a good time to be reminded of this very excellent two-step organizing principle that you may have uttered numerous times yourself. It will save you hours of frustration.

Think about the things you use daily. Where do you keep your house keys? Do you have a place to put a pen and paper by each telephone? What do you do with your purse when you arrive home, or your wallet at night? What about your sunglasses, the dog leash, unpaid bills, your library card, theater tickets? During the coming week, notice what items you need regularly, and then establish a specific place to put those items.

We all have good intentions, but the "for now" attitude often takes over. "I'll just put this here for now . . ." will cost you far more time than the extra moments it would take to get your keys in the drawer, your scarf hung on the hook, or the remote phone back in its cradle. Make a rule: If you take it out, put it away.

"This one is my downfall," says William, who is still active in business. "I've never been a particularly organized person, and I've lost things for days because I didn't put them away and I can't see to find them."

The following organizing principles will also save you time and headaches:

Talk to family members. Everyone from a spouse to visiting children should be made aware that it is crucial that they put away what they have used.

Consider a "lock-up." If the family doesn't put items back in their place, you have to protect yourself. Select a drawer that is a bit out of the way; mark it "Personal" if you need to. Keep the items you really care about there so that you'll always be able to find what you need.

Acquire multiples. For the common tools you use every day, try to acquire duplicates so that you can keep them wherever you use them. Scissors and magnifiers are good examples. Decide where you need certain household tools and then work on collecting extras.

Give family members a list of the utilitarian items you would like to receive as gifts. A broad-brimmed hat in your car as well as in the front closet will enable you to protect your eyes on gray days that turn sunny. Enough staplers to put wherever you do paperwork will be greatly appreciated.

Take advantage of adaptive aids. Adaptive aids are to someone with macular degeneration what a stethoscope is to a doctor—necessary tools. While a large-face or talking watch may seem unstylish at first, you'll soon wonder why you ever did without it. A visit to a low-vision store or a look through a good product catalog (see Resources) will provide you with countless time-saving devices.

Marking and Labeling

Developing a system for relabeling items as you acquire them will simplify everything from putting your hands on the cinnamon to being able to identify first-class postage stamps (as opposed to stamps of lower denominations) based on the way you label the envelope where you keep them.

Many items needn't be labeled because they are recognizable in other ways. When cooking, your nose will quickly tell lemon extract apart from vanilla extract, for example. In your closet, a lace blouse has a different feel from a silk blouse, so you needn't bother to mark it.

Otherwise, shape, color, contrast, and texture are keys to identifying items. While everything can be relabeled in such a way that you can read what it is, your first choice should always be to create ways to identify items right away.

One idea is to store objects in containers of different shapes. By putting one type of salad dressing in a Mason jar and leaving the other in the original bottle, for example, you'll know which is which. Or purposely purchase shampoo in one type of bottle and buy conditioner in another. This principle can be applied in many circumstances.

Multicolor containers are very helpful. Storage container sets are often made to match, but if you watch for them, and shop at flea markets, you will find some containers that let you separate items by color.

Use rubber bands or plastic ties to demarcate some items. If you have a whole milk and a skim milk container in the re-frigerator, try putting a rubber band around one of the cartons to differentiate. Plastic twist ties or pipe cleaners can be used to identify your toothbrush, mark a control on a CD sound system, or mark your favorite paring knife.

When an item needs to be relabeled, you have a wide variety of options: Black felt-tip markers always come in handy, so purchase a dozen of them so you can keep them in drawers located throughout the house. In addition, nail polish, puff paint (a craft item), cork/felt dots (establish a system for using one, two, or three dots to identify something), safety pins, Velcro, or Hi-Mark can all be used. Hi-Mark is a marking liquid that is available at low-vision stores; in addition to being visible, it has texture so you can also detect it by feel. You may have other ideas that work for you.

Masking tape or white labels from an office supply store should be kept wherever you keep your black pens or other marking equipment. While you may be able to write directly onto a bottle or package, you may need to affix tape or a label on the surface first. Also, keep all labeling simple. For example, if you have no other spice that begins with a c, then a big C for cinnamon may be all you need.

Staying organized is a continual process, not a one-time activity. Each day you need to focus on assessing your to-do list, picking up, putting away, and generally maintaining a routine. By doing so, you'll find that the ten minutes you might otherwise have wasted searching for your house keys can now be devoted to reading (or listening to) a little more of that book you're enjoying, or talking on the phone with a friend.

Invest in Helpful Products

Visiting a store or going through a catalog of low-vision products can give you fresh ideas on handy items. You'll find:

- Wristwatches that announce the time when you push a button. Add to that talking calculators, thermostats, Caller ID sets—more talking items than can be mentioned here.
- Oversized timers that are easy to set (and to locate once you've put them down!). You can keep track of cooking times or sprinkler settings, or set the timer as a reminder for when you need to leave for an appointment.
- Large-print items ranging from calendars to dictionaries.
- Needles that you can thread without having to see the eye.
- Large-print games of many types, ranging from Scrabble to backgammon.

See if a low-vision store is located in your area. If not, get on the mailing list of one of the catalogs mentioned in the Resources section.

Help from Others

If you're like many older people, you have what you need. You don't need another pretty new scarf. Another set of dish towels is something you could live without.

Your family has just gotten a whole new lease on birthday and holiday gifts. Now instead of getting one more thing that you didn't really need, you can tell family members new items that really will be useful to you.

Tell them you're going to create a wish list of helpful items. Point out a store in your area where you can purchase useful products, or go through a catalog with them and select items. More and more books are coming out on audio, so for the relative who always enjoyed giving you books, tell them to send you the audio version instead.

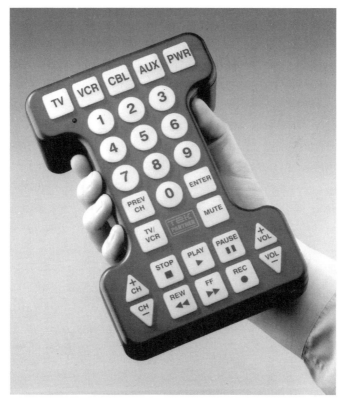

A universal remote control for a television and VCR that features an easy-to-see control panel. *Credit: Lighthouse International*

There's a Learning Curve

Just as your symptoms may ebb and flow to some degree, so, too, will your ability to manage. You'll be learning new skills and new ways to use your senses. You will master these elements, but as with everything else, you will have good days and bad days. If you're exhausted from trying to get your computer program or your reading machine to function properly, remember that frustration was part of your life even before AMD set in. That said, people do report fatigue. On a bad day Ralph's solution is to give himself a break and stay home. "The next day I'll be ready to try again," he says.

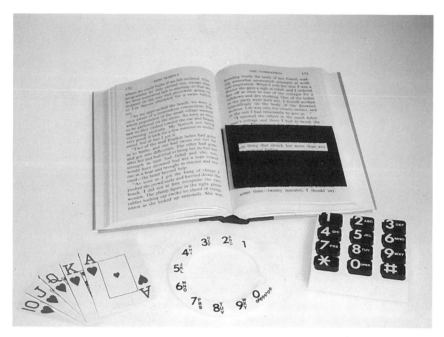

These nonoptical devices are helpful to people with low vision. TOP: A reading guide (typoscope) makes reading easier by isolating a line of type. BOTTOM, LEFT TO RIGHT: playing cards with large faces; large-faced numbers for a rotary dial phone; large-faced numbers for a push-button phone.   *Credit: Lighthouse International*

Ellen's solution is to get out among people: "I call my friend and suggest lunch," she says.

Some days will be more challenging than others. Call someone for help or advice, or consider doing something nice for yourself. Call a friend, or give yourself an afternoon to just putter, not worrying about whether you get anything done.

Adjusting to a new life is an opportunity to toss out the bad parts of the old. If you set priorities, changes can be made for the better. Let's go on to more specific areas in the next few chapters, and find out how useful ideas can become a practical part of your daily life.

10

Your Home Environment

When it comes to your household, think *convenience* and *contrast*.

Convenience means anything from rethinking the furniture arrangement so you can move around freely, to putting items away promptly so that you'll be able to find them the next time you need them.

Using contrast in the home makes everything easier to see. Whether you buy white mugs from which to drink your black coffee or use dark blue towels in a white bathroom, you'll find that contrasting colors will make objects more visible.

Before getting to these, however, there are some important general safety precautions.

- Smoke alarms should be installed and checked regularly. The fire department recommends changing the batteries when you change the clocks for daylight saving time. If a battery wears out in the meantime, a low beep will be emitted regularly. If your smoke alarm should go off, leave the house immediately and call 911 from a neighbor's.

The fire department never minds responding to a false alarm. They live by the creed "Better safe than sorry."

- Have your water heater thermostat adjusted so that it is no higher than 120 degrees. That reduces the risk of scalding.
- Secure scatter rugs with nonskid rug backing or fasten the edges using rug tape.
- In the bathtub or shower stall, use nonskid mats or add decals that provide traction.
- Consider having a safety rail professionally installed in your tub or shower. Don't ever use a soap dish handle or a towel bar as a support rail.
- Toxic substances should be kept in a designated area, and marked in such a way that you know exactly what they are. Anyone else who uses your cleaning liquids or insect sprays should put them away in the appointed place.

Household Navigation

People generally know their own homes so well that they can navigate without additional aids. In a familiar environment, the only danger is when something is out of place. Anyone who comes into your home to visit or to help with housework should be instructed to leave furniture just as they found it and to be vigilant about eliminating clutter, particularly on the floor.

A half-open door, a swinging medicine cabinet mirror, or a kitchen cabinet that is partway open are all extremely hazardous because you may not see them. Get in the habit of leaving doors either open or closed, and closing cabinets the moment you've removed what you need. Make certain others in your home are aware of how important this practice is.

If you have moved, or have difficulty seeing within your house at a specific time of day, here are some additional safety precautions to take. First of all, mark steps and changes in surfaces. Thresholds are hard to see because they blend in. Consider using safety tape or a tread strip to mark these areas.

Next, consider any stairs in your home. Whether it's a full set of stairs or only a step or two, a handrail will provide an extra measure of safety. If there is any chance you could arrive at the top of a staircase without realizing it, think about what you can do to establish a warning cue. Use commercially available safety tape or tread strips to mark the first and last step in a staircase if necessary. (Masking or duct tape sometimes doesn't adhere well and can lift up and catch on your shoe.) Or if you have an unusually steep back staircase or one into the garage that gives you trouble, try using yellow paint to demarcate the edge of the step.

Evaluate furniture located in prime pathways. If an item has sharp edges, you may want to move it. Coffee tables are often hazardous. They are low, often get shifted around by people sitting near them, and can be difficult to see. Moving your coffee table aside is one solution, and establishing contrast is another. Select an area rug that contrasts with the rest of the floor and put the coffee table on the area rug so that it's easily visible.

In the Kitchen

Most kitchens feature good lighting, but you'll be further aided if you have under-the-cabinet lighting. This type of lighting can sometimes be mounted without major electrical work. An adjustable or gooseneck lamp in the kitchen is another way to enhance your kitchen lighting. Being able to check a measurement by holding a cup or a spoon directly beneath a light is a definite help. Be sure, though, your lamp can be placed so that the electrical cord is safely out of the way.

If you use a CCTV reading machine, consider putting it in or near the kitchen. Since the kitchen is the hub of so much activity, having the machine handy means you can slip over to it to check a recipe or a piece of mail.

Some people find mirrors helpful in the kitchen. One woman has mirrors as backsplashes. Not until she got AMD did she realize how helpful the mirrors were in reflecting and amplifying light. Note, however, that this type of lighting may be bothersome to some, so buy an inexpensive household mirror to test this setup before making an investment.

Kitchen Safety

Kitchen safety is of paramount importance. Open upper cabinets, knives, gas flame, and the possibility of breaking a glass all present hazards of particular concern if you have low vision.

- Particularly if you use a gas cooktop, don't wear clothing with loose sleeves that could catch on fire.
- Turn pan handles inward from the counter edge and away from any ON burners where they might become hot.
- Put dishes that will be cooked in the oven on a cookie sheet. It will make retrieval of the hot dish much easier than fishing around in a hot oven.
- Keep an open box of baking soda in a specific spot near the stove in case anything catches on fire, but be prepared to leave the house immediately if the fire involves anything more than a brief spark. The biggest mistake people make is trying to fight a "small" fire themselves.

Call 911. The fire department will make certain the fire doesn't get out of hand.

- If you are concerned about breaking glassware or china, try using plastic dishes and glasses when you can. There are some attractive nonbreakable styles on the market now.
- When handling glassware, use one hand to locate the edge of the counter, and then be certain that the glass is placed well back on the counter.
- Hardware stores sell a specialty knife with a slicing guide. You can adjust the guide to cut different thicknesses.
- Identify a specific drawer for knives and put them away, all facing in the same direction. If you have a dish-washer, put knives point-down in the silverware tray or lay them out on the rack.

Organize

Most people don't take the time to rethink their use of kitchen shelf space—they simply put things away the best they can when they acquire them. Instead, reevaluate. Toss what you don't like and don't use, and put up high the dishes and glasses you use infrequently.

Group foods in your pantry: soup cans in one spot, canned fruit in another, cake mixes separated from other types of boxed mixes. Store your spices near where you use them, and keep only those that you actually use. You may find labeling the shelves easier than relabeling items.

Fresh items in the refrigerator should be both labeled and organized. When you arrive home from the grocery store, take self-adhesive labels (or tape) and a black felt-tip pen and relabel all items with expiration dates. Then arrange the food on refrigerator shelves so that the oldest items are the most accessible. The current milk is moved to the front while the brand-new milk is placed toward the back.

Store your most frequently used items in the most accessible places, and store the rest of the plates and glasses in a less accessible cabinet. You'll still have them if you have company, but they won't clutter up what you need day-to-day.

Finally, get in the habit of putting away what you've used.

Use Contrast

If you have dark counters, use white dishes. If you have light counters, invest in dark dinnerware. Outlet covers and light switches that contrast with the wall will make finding them easier.

If your cabinets have dark interiors, consider having them painted white inside, or put light-colored contact paper on the back wall of the cabinet. One weekend I put down white rubber shelf liners in my mother's dark cabinets and tried to put contact paper on the back of the cabinets. The rubber mats worked well, but the paper came down over time. However, she decided to get the cabinets painted after she realized what a difference a white interior made!

Setting Dials

Use a Velcro or felt square, a dot of nail polish or puff paint to mark your oven dials. The ON position should be marked, and then place a dot at 350°. If you need to cook anything at a higher or a lower temperature, you can adjust from there. (Too many markings will be confusing.)

The keypads of electronic ovens and microwaves are virtually impossible to read because of the way the numbers are stenciled onto the front of the appliance with nothing to demarcate the separate number keys. Low-vision stores and catalogs sell high-contrast stick-on numbers that will permit you to see the key controls.

Measuring

Specialty catalogs sell measuring cups with easy-to-read markings. However, if, like many others with AMD, you have been using the same measuring cups for fifteen to twenty years, you may find that simply purchasing a new cup with bright new markings will solve your problem.

If you use cups in various gradations (1/4, 1/3, 1/2, etc.) for measuring, create your own marking system. Use nail polish or Hi-Mark to write the measuring quantities on the handle of each cup. You can also run a finger along the top edge of the cup to feel when the cup is full, or a simple cork can be invaluable: Put your hand over the top of the cup while pouring slowly; when you feel the cork rise to the top, you know the cup is almost full. Specialty catalogs sell a gadget called Say When that serves a similar purpose.

General Tips

If any of your appliances are wearing out, consider color and contrast when you shop for a new one. Are the knobs easy to use, and do they contrast with the appliance? Ask the appliance store for instruction manuals on cassette. A good number of the major companies have created manuals in large print and braille, and many provide audio instructions.

Many people find that toaster ovens and microwaves are easier to use than a regular stove. Once you know a setting for heating tea in the microwave, the process is much safer.

Always use a timer when cooking. This will ensure that your food is adequately cooked, and it will prevent you from forgetting about something on the stove. Also, use an oven mitt instead of a hot pad. It will protect you from burns on your wrist or hands.

In the Bathroom

One handy bathroom tip is to select towels that contrast with the rest of the bathroom decor. A dark blue towel and washcloth in a white bathroom will be easier to see. Bath mats can be selected the same way. Make sure to use a rubber-backed mat to prevent slipping.

If you've raised children, you may remember that the safest way to run a bath or start a shower is to start out with the cold water and add the hot slowly. When you're finished, turn off the hot first. Check the water temperature with your hand before getting in.

If you take baths, put a dot or a mark of some type at the level you prefer. When the water reaches that point, you'll know to turn off the faucets. Or float a brightly colored sponge in the tub—as it rises, you'll know where the water level is.

Here are a few more ideas:

- A contrasting color of soap, soap-on-a-rope, or soap in colored netting is enormously handy.
- Keep some type of magnifying lens in the bathroom so that you can check medicine labels and instructions.
- A magnifying mirror on a stand or on an arm that attaches to and swings out from the wall can be useful for shaving or applying makeup.

In Your Closet

You should have a light installed in the closet if you don't already have one. Also keep a flashlight on a convenient shelf so that you'll have added light when you need it.

Much of your clothing will be easily recognized by touch, but organize clothing by type: casual slacks at one end of the rod, dress slacks at the other, etc. Some people like to organize sets of clothing. For example, if you have a tie that looks best with a certain suit, hang that tie on the hanger with that suit.

Establish a sign system to identify colors. Use index cards with "Brown" written in large letters, or cut the index card into a shape—circles mark all black things; triangles mark navy blue, etc. Punch a hole in the card or the top of the shape and attach this to the appropriate hanger. Also, when an item is sent to the cleaner, pull the hanger out of the regular part of your closet so that when the clothing is returned, you can rehang it on the correct hanger.

People with little or no vision use a code system for more permanently marking their clothing, and you may want to do this with some items that are more difficult to identify. Use different-shaped buttons or small safety pins and create a code. Note your code on a master list so you'll have a way to keep track of your labeling system. No pin on a shirt might indicate white; one pin fastened horizontally, blue; one pin fastened vertically, black; two pins crossed, red. Be sure the buttons or pins are placed inside the garment in such a way that they aren't uncomfortable.

In drawers, you can use dividers to separate items for easier identification. In addition, try using sock sorters (clips that hold together a pair of socks) in the laundry. If you clip together a pair of black socks, you're sure to have them correctly paired when they come out of the wash.

With some minor adjustments, you'll soon find that your home can be everything you've always wanted it to be—comfortable, convenient, and, of course, safe.

This chapter contains the more commonly used ideas for organizing. Be creative and think of some on your own. You may discover a hidden talent you never knew you had.

11

Simple Systems for Daily Tasks

"If I make the routine parts of my day as simple as possible, it leaves me more energy for doing something new or different," says Katherine. "It just pays to streamline and simplify."

As you begin, you may want to see how well you are keeping track of your life. First off, check your calendar and your address book. Are these big enough so that you can write in large enough letters to comfortably see what you've written? If your calendar system or address book is pocket-size, you may want to switch to something larger.

For an ongoing to-do list, consider using a three-ring binder if you need more space. A loose-leaf notebook's ample size allows you to write as large as you need to without feeling squeezed. If you select one of the thin ones with a plastic cover, the notebook will be light enough to take with you. If the notebook is still bigger than you want to carry, you can transfer each day's to-do items onto large index cards, writing down one task on each card. You can note down everything from a reminder to buy a birthday card for a friend to a list of questions you want to ask the ophthalmologist.

When you purchase your notebook and paper, invest in dividers with pockets. Though the thin binders will hold only one or two dividers, this still provides you with one or two pockets to store support materials for the items on your list. For example, the ticket for the watch that is in for repair could be kept in one pocket. The insurance letter you want to discuss with your daughter in another.

Once you're set up, write everything down. Again, this applies to all people of all ages—why bother to remember things when you can note them down as reminders for later?

Check your calendar and notebook daily. Make certain you establish the habit of checking for appointments and items that need doing. As you scan through the notebook each morning, cross off the items you accomplished the day before.

The Telephone

Local telephone companies provide a variety of services for consumers with special needs.

Directory Exemption. This service permits those who have registered with the phone company to be exempt from 411 (directory information) charges.

Operator Assistance. The operator will dial a number for you at no charge.

Voice-activated dialing system. The system dials for you based on the number you tell it orally. Some companies are beginning to offer this service, and an increasing number will in the future because of the popularity of car phones and the need of the general population to have hands-free methods of talking on the telephone.

Call your local phone company to learn what is available in your area. In addition, here are some other conveniences that may help you use the telephone:

Speed-dial numbers are a big help if you have a phone that can be programmed for you. Program in emergency numbers as well. Also, look for caller IDs that give audio readouts of who has called.

Next to each telephone, keep a directory that provides information large enough for you to read. Large-format address/telephone books are also available commercially. If your directory is in the computer, print out a copy that is in a large-size font; if your numbers aren't computerized, then when friends or family members say, "What can I do to help?" you have the perfect job for them—hand copying your telephone directory using larger, blacker printing.

In the future, phones will feature some sort of tactile demarcation of the buttons. My current phone has a slight bump on the number 5, which makes dialing easier since I can easily identify the center number on the touch-tone pad.

In an emergency, dial 0 for the operator. If you are feeling flustered, this is as sure a method of getting help as trying to dial 911.

Medications

Establishing some type of marking system—from black writing on the label to tactile shapes glued to the bottle—for your medications is very important. You may be groggy one day when you get up to take your medicine, and you want to be sure of exactly what you are taking.

In addition to labeling the medications you take regularly, go through the rest of your medicine cabinet. Toss what you no longer take, and label miscellaneous treatments like cold remedies and anti-itch creams. Though organizing your medicines takes time, you can make relabeling them when purchased part of the process of putting them away. Note what it is, how much to take, and what the expiration date is. If you use one of the CCTV machines, take all medications to the machine and do your assessment there.

Nancy Paskin of Lighthouse International recommends a good system for anyone managing medications that are to be taken more than once each day: Put on the bottle the number of rubber bands that represents the dosage you are to take throughout the day (three rubber bands for something to be taken three times per day). Each time you take the medicine, remove one of the rubber bands. At the end of the day, replace the rubber bands.

Also, if you know the color and texture of any pills that you are taking, this will help prevent taking the wrong pill at the wrong time.

Money

Being able to identify money is crucial to getting along well with less vision. While the newly released bills with larger numbers and larger images are a definite help, the United States is not yet as advanced as some foreign countries, where the bills are in different colors and even different sizes.

To be certain what denomination of bill you are handing someone, consider using a wallet that has various sections. Then you can separate your bills at home and place various denominations in different sections of the wallet.

Other people use a folding system:

$1—place unfolded in your wallet.
$5—fold the five-dollar bill in half, short ends together.
$10—fold the ten in half, long sides together.
$20—fold this bill in half and then in half again.

Coins can be identified by touch. The sizes of the coins are all different, and pennies and nickels have smooth edges while dimes and quarters have ridged edges. Use your fingernail along the edge of the coin if you need to double-check.

When paying for something, try to hand the cashier the bill that is closest to the amount of the sale. State the bill that you're putting out, and ask the cashier to identify the bills given you in return.

Paying Bills

In today's busy world, there are several ways you can simplify your life so that you needn't spend a lot of time writing checks. Just as you can direct-deposit income checks, you can also authorize certain bill payments. With your permission, your bank will automatically pay your mortgage and phone and utility bills. Talk to an officer of the bank to see if there are other payments that might be streamlined.

In addition, consolidate your bills when you can. Rather than using several different credit cards, select one bank card and try to put most of your charges on it. That way at the end of the month you will review fewer bills and will have to write fewer checks.

Check Signing and Writing by Hand

Some people write checks using the flatbed of their CCTV reading machine. By placing the check on the flatbed, they are then able to see the places that need to be filled in.

A special check-writing device is available from catalogs and specialty stores. The template is set on the check itself, and spaces are left for each of the areas where you need to write something—the date, to whom the check is written, the

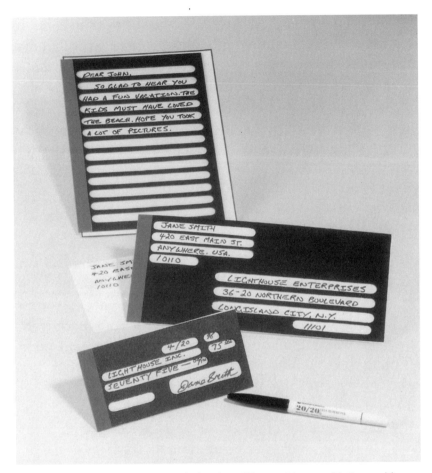

Here are some examples of check-writing guides and letter-writing guides, available from low-vision centers and catalogs.
Credit: Lighthouse International

amount, and your signature. By moving the template from check to check you can easily pay your own bills. Checks are also available with raised markings (ridges where the lines are) so that you can feel the format of the check to fill it out properly.

To sign documents, there are several workable methods. You can have someone use a black felt-tip pen to darken the line on which you're to sign, for instance. Or ask them to place a Post-it note right along the line to be signed. You'll be able to feel the ridge of the note and sign on top of that. Another method is to have someone place the index finger of your non-writing hand in the place where you are to sign. This will guide you as to where to sign.

For writing letters by hand, you can purchase specialty paper with bold lines. This along with a felt-tip pen can give you the guidance you need. Letter-writing guides (like check-writing templates) are also available. If it's hard to see where the writing paper ends, place it on a contrasting surface.

Eating

Color contrast can be as important with food on the plate as it is with the plate on the mat. If possible, serve dark food on a light plate and light food on a dark one. You may find that patterned dishes are problematic. It's difficult to find the green beans if you're looking at plate with vines painted all over it.

If you're confused about exactly what is on the plate, ask the person you're with to describe the location of the food using the clock method. (What's at six o'clock? What's at two o'clock?) If you're alone or don't want to ask, use your fork to gently probe the food to see what you have and where it is.

If you're serving yourself at the kitchen counter, get in the habit of putting foods in specific places on the plate. As you carry the plate to the table, hold it in the same position it was in while on the counter. When you put it down, you'll know where the various servings were placed.

As you eat, work inward on the plate. This will help you locate the food and lessen the likelihood of pushing food onto the table.

Foods like peas are very difficult for anyone to eat. Now that you're having vision problems you can be inventive about it. Use a piece of bread, a roll, or even the edge of a spoon or knife to push the food onto your fork.

Cutting food can be done by feel, but if you're eating at a restaurant, you may feel less stressed if you order a pasta dish (probably not spaghetti!) or a white fish dish that doesn't require much cutting.

To identify the salt shaker, feel them both. Salt is heavier than pepper. To avoid overseasoning, pour either condiment into the palm of your hand and sprinkle just a pinch over your food.

Remember contrast. Buy a white cup if you're a coffee drinker, for example, and serve drinks in a distinctive color of glass.

At a restaurant or someone's home, the whereabouts of your water may be a mystery, so you'll want to employ the "sweep" method, which can be done discreetly. Use the side of your hand (or arm if there are no dishes on the table yet) to sweep slowly across the surface of the table in front of you. You'll quickly locate the base of your glass. Because the movement is subtle, no one need be aware of how many times you must go on a "glass hunt."

To pour liquids, try putting the glass or cup on a tray with edges. If you spill, the liquid will be contained.

If you're pouring something cold from a pitcher, use your fingers to position the spout over the glass, and then let your index finger (placed inside the inner edge of the glass) be your guide.

With hot liquids, you need to be careful not to get burned. By paying careful attention, you may be able to fill the cup simply by feeling the warmth emanating to the outside of the cup. Stop when you feel it rising. As when filling measuring cups, you can use a cork or other commercially available gadgets that float to the top and tell you when your cup is full.

Personal Grooming

Brushing your teeth probably isn't hard with AMD, but getting the toothpaste on the brush might be. Shop for a toothbrush made of colored plastic instead of clear. Or try placing your toothbrush on a contrasting-colored washcloth to make the brush and the paste more visible. Or place your index finger along the edges of the bristles, letting your finger serve as a guide for the paste.

For both shaving and applying makeup, a simple magnifying mirror or a lighted one on a stand may be very helpful. When shaving, work systematically. You've always done it by feel; you've just used your eyesight as a "crutch." Then, as you complete each area, use your free hand to check for any missed spots.

As for applying makeup, plan a simple system that achieves the look you want without requiring a lot of products. Store these in a compartmentalized unit or a small basket so that items are easy to locate. For the first couple of weeks, have your spouse or the friend you're meeting do a quick check—after that, you'll likely have it down pat. Along the same lines, consult with a hair stylist or barber for a hairstyle that's easy to maintain.

Being Methodical Can Save the Day

At Lighthouse International, rehabilitation teachers, led by Nancy Paskin, teach three basic steps for accomplishing a specific task—from wiping a kitchen counter to shaving.

1. Define the area. Break large areas into manageable sections, defined by certain landmarks.
2. Use overlapping strokes to be certain you don't miss anything. After you finish one area (for example, in

shaving), move over only slightly, so that the next stroke partially overlaps the preceding one.

3. Check your work, correcting anything that needs to be redone.

You can also apply this three-step method when you can't locate something (see below for further suggestions).

Here's another example of a task that will become easier with this orderly process: mowing the lawn.

When you go outside, first set up a radio as an auditory cue to locate a certain landmark—the porch or garage, perhaps, or whatever works best for you.

Wear safety glasses—tinted ones for sun or glare protection. Then walk along the first section to be mowed, picking up branches and twigs that could be obstacles. If needed, use bricks or some type of specific obstacle to mark flower beds so that you can locate the edge of the grass. As you do in shaving, work systemically, overlapping your rows so that you are sure all the grass gets cut.

When You Can't Find Something

Earlier we discussed the importance of the organizing principle "A place for everything and everything in its place." Yet we all know that "real life" happens: the phone or the doorbell rings, and you put something down. Later you haven't a clue what you did with it. Of course, this happens to people with perfect vision, too. Finding a missing item is that much more difficult if your sight isn't perfect, so what you need is strategies.

Systematic searches are the way to locate something that's missing. Whether it's retracing every inch you traveled when you came in the door, in search of your house keys (be sure to check whether they're still in the outer door), or feeling your way through every shelf in the refrigerator looking for leftovers, begin at a specified starting point and work from there. You'll soon find whatever you lost.

In order to recover a dropped object, listen to determine where the item falls in relation to where you are. If you've dropped the item on the carpet, there may have been no sound, so check the area near your shoes and between your feet. Before bending down, be certain you're not standing near something that could hit your head on the way down. (The same is true for standing up if you find you must crawl around a bit in search of the item.) Turn and face the direction in which you think the object fell. Search systematically using your hands, until you've covered the area from your feet to arm's length. Items bounce, so if you don't find something in the direction in which you think it fell, search the area behind you.

A broom can be very helpful as well. Sweep the area of the floor where you think the item was dropped. Sweep systematically and sweep to a specific point. Now you can search a reduced area; with luck the broom will pick up the item and bring it within range.

If you have trouble bending, use your feet to locate larger items. If you need to bend down, use a counter or table to provide balance and go down slowly.

Here's another idea. For a small item, an item dropped on carpet, or one you don't want to mix in with dust, use a ruler. Lay it flat on the floor and slowly fan left and right. This technique allows you to cover a larger area, though if there are pieces of furniture, you'll locate their legs as well.

Don't be overly discouraged about dropping something. If it's not hazardous, wait until someone is around to help you search. If you remember dropping a nail or an earring when your eyes were just fine, you'll know that dropped items do mysterious things. It may take even a fully sighted person a couple of searches to find it. (Grandkids are great at this task.)

Though at times tasks may take longer than you might like, everything will get better with practice. Keep working at what's important to you. You may even discover some "secrets" that will make certain tasks easier than they've ever been.

A Little Humor Helps in a Big Way

When all else fails and you've just appeared on the street wearing one black shoe and one brown shoe, try calling up your sense of humor. People with macular degeneration laugh at their own stories of wearing mismatched socks or returning to the wrong table at a restaurant. One woman even chuckles about the day she entered the men's room by accident.

12

Can I Still Drive?

"I can't imagine not driving."

"I'll be so depressed if I can't go where I want when I want."

"I'll lose my independence if I can't drive."

If you live anywhere except in a major city with a good public transit system, then you are very concerned about how much longer you'll be able to drive. To Americans, the ability to get around by car signifies freedom and independence to such a level that people with many types of physical changes fight hard to maintain their ability to continue driving an automobile.

This chapter explains the legal requirements necessary to maintain a license and offers advice on how to remain a good driver for as long as possible after a diagnosis of AMD. For many the day will come when driving is no longer a good idea. When you can no longer see well enough to be sure you will **always** notice a child following a ball into the street or a pedestrian crossing in front of you if there is glare, it is vital that you listen to your own instincts or the recommendations of loved ones who feel it is time for you to look for alternative ways to get around. This chapter also provides suggestions of new ways to get where you need to go every day.

Many patients with AMD are legally qualified to drive and have the capability of being good drivers. Unfortunately, the vision test conducted by the Department of Motor Vehicles is really not indicative of who can see well enough to drive, and many people do not test well under stressful circumstances. Nerves, the hectic bureaucratic environment, or an impatient state employee can all have an effect on your ability to do well on the test.

If a vision test is required for an upcoming license renewal, drivers with AMD are best served by picking up a form to be filled out by their eye doctor. In addition to conducting the required tests, an eye-care professional can make recommendations that will help you see the road better while driving. Your glasses may require adjustment, and many drivers find that tinted lenses of a specific hue can heighten contrast. Ultimately, you and your eye-care professional must also agree that you still see well enough to react when the unexpected happens—the absolute key to safe driving.

Qualifying for License Renewal

Minimum vision requirements for driving vary from state to state. Most states have a two-part vision requirement, one for visual acuity and one for measurement of a person's visual field.

Visual Acuity

Visual acuity is your ability to discern objects from a distance, and it is tested by assessing your ability to read an eye chart. In most states corrected acuity for driving (meaning that you are permitted to wear glasses for the testing) is generally set at 20/20 to 20/40. If you no longer meet the criteria for driving in your state, talk to your eye-care specialist. He or she may be able to provide you with lenses that will allow you to drive for a little longer.

Visual Field

The visual field test measures your ability to use your side or peripheral vision. Generally this is not a problem for someone with macular degeneration since the disease primarily affects central vision.

The test is designed to assess how much you see of a full panoramic view of the world (180 degrees). Each eye is tested separately. You can check your visual field yourself by conducting a simple test.

To test the right side, put your right arm straight in front of you with your fingers level with your eyes. Cover the left eye with your left hand, and look straight ahead with the right eye. Throughout the test, the right eye should continue to look straight ahead. Now move your right arm (the outstretched one) to the right so that it is straight out to your side at shoulder level. Using your side vision (since your eye is still focused forward), can you still see your fingertips? If so, your peripheral vision to the right is 90 degrees.

Still with your right arm extended, move it in an arc back across your body at shoulder height, left eye closed and right one focused straight ahead. You are considered to have normal peripheral vision if you can still see your fingertips as your right arm crosses over your body as far as it can go (probably so that your right fingers are even with your left shoulder), giving you a visual field of approximately 110 degrees with the right eye.

To test the visual field on the other side, repeat with your left eye.

If both eyes test well, you have a visual field of 180 degrees.

Officially, a measurement of visual field is made on a "perimeter." In this simple test the doctor has you look at a target while an object is brought in from the side. The doctor then records the visual field horizontally, vertically, and diagonally.

When Full Licenses Must Be Limited

Getting a Restricted License

In some states, eye-care professionals are given the power to determine if a patient who doesn't qualify for a full license is capable of driving under certain conditions. The possibilities for a restricted license are quite broad. A doctor may specify only in good weather; only during daylight, not at dawn or dusk (because of glare); on local streets only; between the hours of 9 A.M. and 3 P.M., etc. A required reexamination date is usually specified on a restricted license.

Bioptic Glasses with a Restricted License

Restricted licenses that permit driving with "bioptic telescope glasses," special glasses for low-vision drivers, can be issued under special circumstances.

These glasses have prescription lenses in their lower portion. This is known as the "carrier" portion of the eyeglass, through which a driver views the road. The upper portion of the better eye is fitted with a small self-focusing telescope. Think of them as bifocals with a telescope in the upper section of one of the lenses. The telescope serves as a "spotting" device to be used for quick peeks at items such as street signs or stoplights that are too far away for a person with AMD to see with normal glasses. The bioptic glasses do not make seeing the road or oncoming traffic any easier. They correct vision only for faraway items.

More than half the states now allow telescopic devices for people who need them. However, many of these states require that drivers retake the driving portion of the test in order to be certified for driving with these glasses.

Use of bioptic glasses requires special training and practice, and obtaining them is a three-step process:

1. Your low-vision specialist will prescribe and fit you for them.
2. The specialist or another rehabilitation specialist will train you to use the glasses.
3. You will need special driver's training. Ask about this at your low-vision center, or contact the Association of Drivers Educators for the Disabled. This organization can put you in touch with a qualified instructor in your area who can work with you on the use of the bioptic glasses before driving. Working with a driving teacher who understands the use of the glasses is preferable. However, because finding anyone with the proper training is often difficult, many bioptic drivers train under a regular driving instructor. If you have already received some training from your low-vision specialist, a regular driving school can provide you with someone who will help you refine your driving technique while using the device. Check the telephone book for driving schools in your area.

Mark, an audio engineer in his mid-thirties who uses bioptic glasses to drive, puts this aid in perspective: "Driving is really important to me, so I'm glad I've had the option of bioptic glasses, but it's a lot of work. It requires great concentration and a high level of general awareness of the road."

Check the charts below and on the following pages to see if driving with bioptic glasses is permitted in your state.

State	Visual acuity	Visual field	Special license	Bioptic telescopes
Alabama	20/40 UR	Horizontal temporal visual field of 110 unrestricted	20/60 (cutoff) <110 restricted based on vision specialist's recommendation	N/A
Alaska	20/40 UR	Visual field only with a telescopic lens: 60 (cutoff) to 90 degrees; < than 60 degrees not licensed until VA requirements can be met without lenses	20/50–20/100 cutoff restricted per department review	Allowed but requires side mirrors
Arizona	20/40 UR	60 degrees temporal and 35 nasal	20/50–20/60 daylight only	N/A
Arkansas	20/40	145 degrees for two eyes or 105 for one eye	20/50 with bioptic telescopic	Allowed
California	20/40 better eye 20/67 worse eye	Horizontal field of at least 75 degrees each eye	Same requirement when using a bioptic	Allowed
Colorado	20/40 UR	N/A	20/40 through bioptic	Allowed

UR = unrestricted. There are no restrictions placed on your license
Horizontal temporal field = visual field out to the side
NA = not allowed
Monocular (mono) = one eye
Binocular (bino) = using two eyes
The authors thank Lori L. Grover, OD, FAAO, and Terra Barnes, OD, FAAO, for the data on pp. 168–178.

State	Visual acuity	Visual field	Special license	Bioptic telescopes
Connecticut	20/40 UR	140 degrees binocular and 100 degrees monocular	N/A	NA
Delaware	20/40 UR	N/A	Between 20/40 and 20/70 restricted; < 20/50 denied pending approval from Medical Advisory board	Bioptic drivers evaluated on an individual basis
District of Columbia	N/A	N/A	N/A	Bioptic can be used
Kentucky	20/40 UR	110 degrees; if less referred to medical board	With bioptic: 120 degree horizontal and 80 vertical field; 20/60 through bioptic	Bioptics allowed; 20/200 or better
Louisiana	20/40 UR	N/A	20/50–20/70 may get limited privileges; 20/80–20/100 must pass driving test; <20/100 referred to Conviction/ Medical unit	Not allowed

UR = unrestricted. There are no restrictions placed on your license
Horizontal temporal field = visual field out to the side
NA = not allowed
Monocular (mono) = one eye
Binocular (bino) = using two eyes

State	Visual acuity	Visual field	Special license	Bioptic telescopes
Maine	20/40 UR	140 degree UR	20/70 restricted; 140–110 degree (cutoff) restrictions	Not allowed
Maryland	20/40	140 degrees of field, and binocular vision (simultaneously) for unrestricted	Restricted to side mirrors: 20/40 and 110 field with at least 35 lateral to midline each side; restricted to mirrors and daylight only: 20/70–20/100 and 110 field with 35 lateral to midline with both eyes	Bioptic allowed At 20/100 through the carrier lens, 20/70 through the bioptic, and 150 degrees horizontal for daytime only; after one year—if sees 20/40 through scope and has field, can apply for unrestricted
Minnesota	20/40 UR	N/A	20/50–20/70 restricted; horizontal field 105 degrees unrestricted; less may require restriction(s)	N/A

UR = unrestricted. There are no restrictions placed on your license
Horizontal temporal field = visual field out to the side
NA = not allowed
Monocular (mono) = one eye
Binocular (bino) = using two eyes

State	Visual acuity	Visual field	Special license	Bioptic telescopes
Michigan	20/50 UR	140 degrees	Less than 20/50–20/70 daylight only with no eye disease; 20/50 unrestricted to 20/60 daylight only with eye disease; visual field 140 to 110 unrestricted; less than 110 to 90 subject to restrictions; less than 90 not eligible; 20/100 or less one eye and 20/50 other eye unrestricted; less than 20/50 other eye not eligible	Bioptic: 20/40 through scope and at least 20/100 through the carrier
Mississippi	20/40 right and left eye UR	N/A	20/40 one eye or less subject to restrictions	Allowed

UR = unrestricted. There are no restrictions placed on your license
Horizontal temporal field = visual field out to the side
NA = not allowed
Monocular (mono) = one eye
Binocular (bino) = using two eyes

State	Visual acuity	Visual field	Special license	Bioptic telescopes
Missouri	20/40 UR	55 degrees unrestricted	20/41–20/160 (cutoff); field 85 degrees one eye and unknown other: side mirror	Bioptic can be worn as a supplement to drive but cannot be used to meet 20/160 acuity requirement
Montana	20/40 UR	N/A	20/40–20/70 restricted; 20/70–20/100 suspended, then can request licensure pending approval from regional manager and restrictions from same	N/A
Nebraska	20/40 UR	140 unrestricted	20/40–20/70 (cutoff) one eye and/or other eye, restrictions apply; 100–139 restrictions; cutoff less than 100	Bioptic: can be used and restrictions are determined by examining personnel

UR = unrestricted. There are no restrictions placed on your license
Horizontal temporal field = visual field out to the side
NA = not allowed
Monocular (mono) = one eye
Binocular (bino) = using two eyes

State	Visual acuity	Visual field	Special license	Bioptic telescopes
Nevada	20/40 UR	140 degrees binocular unrestricted	110–140 restrictions	Bioptic: 20/40 through scope; 20/120 through carrier; 130 degrees field; pass road test
New Hampshire	20/40 UR	N/A	20/50–20/70	N/A
New Jersey	20/50 UR	N/A	20/60–20/70	Allowed
New Mexico	20/40 UR	120 degrees total in horizontal meridian	20/50–20/80 (cutoff) restricted; other licensure; up to medical or vision doctor	N/A
New York	20/40 UR	N/A	Visual field of 140 degrees if VA is between 20/40 and 20/70	Bioptic: 20/40 through bioptic VF 140 degrees; with restrictions

UR = unrestricted. There are no restrictions placed on your license
Horizontal temporal field = visual field out to the side
NA = not allowed
Monocular (mono) = one eye
Binocular (bino) = using two eyes

State	Visual acuity	Visual field	Special license	Bioptic telescopes
North Carolina	20/40 monocular 20/50 binocular	N/A	20/50–20/70 monocular; 20/60–20/100 binocular restrictions; field 60 degrees in one eye or 30 on each side of point of fixation	Bioptic cannot be used to meet visual acuity require- ments but can be worn when driving
North Dakota	20/40 UR; 20/30 monocular unrestricted	140 degree UR	20/50–20/100 restrictions; VF 10–120 degrees (cutoff) restrictions; if monocular hori- zontal 120 degrees and vertical 70 degrees	Bioptic: 20/40 through the telescope and 20/130 through carrier
Ohio	20/40 UR	N/A	20/50–20/70 daylight; VF 70 degrees temporal and 45 nasal horizontal	Bioptic: 20/40 through bioptic and no carrier minimum; same field require- ments

UR = unrestricted. There are no restrictions placed on your license
Horizontal temporal field = visual field out to the side
NA = not allowed
Monocular (mono) = one eye
Binocular (bino) = using two eyes

State	Visual acuity	Visual field	Special license	Bioptic telescopes
Oklahoma	20/60 both eyes or 20/50 monocular UR	N/A	VF 70 degrees temporal and 35 nasal at least one eye (cutoff 30 degrees to the right and 30 to left)	Bioptic cannot be worn and bioptic wearers cannot be licensed
Oregon	20/40 UR	N/A	20/50–20/70 daylight unless vision specialist's opinion says otherwise; field 110 degrees minimum	Bioptic can be worn only if vision require-ments are met viewing through carrier lens
Pennsylvania	20/40 unrestricted	N/A	20/60–20/100 restrictions as per vision specialist; field at least 120 degrees in horizontal meridian	N/A
Rhode Island	20/40 UR	115 degrees binocular; 75 temporal and 40 nasal monocular	N/A	N/A

UR = unrestricted. There are no restrictions placed on your license
Horizontal temporal field = visual field out to the side
NA = not allowed
Monocular (mono) = one eye
Binocular (bino) = using two eyes

State	Visual acuity	Visual field	Special license	Bioptic telescopes
South Carolina	20/40 UR	N/A	20/50–20/70 (cutoff) restrictions as per vision specialist	Bioptics can be worn but vision requirements must be met through carriers only
South Dakota	20/40 UR	N/A	20/50–20/60 restrictions; less than 20/60 denied	N/A
Tennessee	20/30 UR	150 degrees in horizontal meridian	20/40–20/70 restricted	20/60 through telescope; 20/200 through carrier; per recommendation of vision specialist/ advisory board
Texas	20/40 UR	N/A	20/70 restricted	Bioptic users must see greater than 20/100 through the carrier
Utah	20/40 UR	120 degrees in the horizontal and 20 degrees vertical	N/A	N/A

UR = unrestricted. There are no restrictions placed on your license
Horizontal temporal field = visual field out to the side
NA = not allowed
Monocular (mono) = one eye
Binocular (bino) = using two eyes

State	Visual acuity	Visual field	Special license	Bioptic telescopes
Vermont	20/40 UR	60 degrees temporal and nasal	N/A	Allowed
Virginia	20/40 UR	100 degrees of horizontal vision UR	N/A	Bioptic: 20/200 through carrier and 20/70 through scope and 70 degrees daylight only one year, then may apply to remove restriction
Washington	20/40 UR	110 degrees	20/50–20/80 restrictions per vision specialist: VF if less than 110 degrees restrictions by vision-care specialist	Bioptics can be used as recommended by vision care specialist
West Virginia	20/40 UR	Not specified	Other referred for examination and report must be approved by Driver's License Advisory Board	N/A

UR = unrestricted. There are no restrictions placed on your license
Horizontal temporal field = visual field out to the side
NA = not allowed
Monocular (mono) = one eye
Binocular (bino) = using two eyes

State	Visual acuity	Visual field	Special license	Bioptic telescopes
Wisconsin	20/40 UR	Horizontal temporal field of at lest 20 degrees or more from center in one eye	20/50–20/200 (cutoff) may require restrictions	Biopic cannot be used to meet acuity require-ments
Wyoming	20/40 UR	N/A	Less than 20/40 may require re-strictions per review of De-partment	Bioptic may be used per recommen-dation of vision specialist

UR = unrestricted. There are no restrictions placed on your license
Horizontal temporal field = visual field out to the side
NA = not allowed
Monocular (mono) = one eye
Binocular (bino) = using two eyes

Qualifying to Drive Is Only the First Step

Once you've been diagnosed with AMD, you've been handed a warning ticket, so to speak. It is vital that you review safe driving guidelines and take your responsibility very seriously, for your own safety and the safety of those around you.

A good driver has the visual ability to perceive change in a rapidly shifting environment, the mental ability to judge what is happening, and the motor skills and flexibility to react quickly and execute the decision. The stronger you keep these other skills, the longer you can continue to drive.

The AARP offers a "55 Alive, Mature Driving" course, available throughout the country. It is an eight-hour course, taught in two four-hour sessions. Cost is minimal—just $10 at this writing. There are no tests. Many people take it to qualify for a discount on their insurance, but a refresher course on safe driving and defensive driving skills is helpful to a driver of any age and ability. Call the AARP for more information, or check their Web site (www.aarp.org).

All drivers will soon benefit from enlarged road signs, mandated by the federal government in 1997. The law allows for a gradual changeover to signs that require six-inch letters for all street names—two inches taller than previously. Municipalities have until 2012 to put up the new signs, but drivers should begin to see some changes in all areas of the country, which should help you feel more comfortable about driving.

Safety First

In addition to AMD-related vision difficulties, older drivers may have more difficulty focusing, which affects their ability to judge distances and speed. Here is some basic driving advice that will be even more important now:

First of all, drive one car consistently. If you need to honk the horn or defog your windshield, you will be able to do so easily because you know where all the controls are. If for some reason you must drive someone else's car, study the dashboard for a few minutes before starting the motor. Identify how to switch on the lights, run the windshield wipers, turn on the heater and defog, and note where the turn signal is.

You should keep your car in good working order. Befriend a local service station owner who will make sure you have everything from excellent tires to clean windshield wiper blades.

You might consider putting in a wider in-car rearview mirror (sold at auto accessory shops). A broader view of the traffic behind the car appeals to restricted and nonrestricted drivers alike.

Keep your windshield clean at all times, both inside and out. It will make a big difference in your ability to see. Also, if your car is dirty, so are your headlights. Make certain the headlights get cleaned even if you don't wash the car. Dirt can reduce light output by 70 percent. In addition to keeping the headlights clean, ask a mechanic to check the aim of your headlights twice a year.

If light hitting the dashboard reflects back onto your windshield and the glare inhibits you from seeing the road, place a black cloth over the dashboard. Tape it carefully along the edge of the windshield and cut and tape the cloth so that it doesn't interfere with your view of the instruments or your use of the controls on the front console. The fabric will absorb the glare.

Of course, seeing well means ensuring optimum vision. Earlier in the book, we discussed how to find your blind spot. Knowing its location, and how to see around it, can be critical to good driving. If you know you have more difficulty seeing things to your right, for example, then you will need to look right more frequently than you used to. Start practicing long before you get behind the wheel. Try sitting on your front porch and looking in the distance. Experiment to find what type of scanning helps bring in the full picture clearly. Next, ask someone else to drive and try this scanning technique when riding as a front-seat passenger. Making a habit of careful scanning is all the more important because a moving car is constantly entering into a changing panorama.

You'll also want to have your eyes checked regularly, and talk to your eye doctor about your driving. Your eye-care professional can keep you fitted with appropriate lenses. One thing to discuss is tinted lenses. If you need help in heightening contrast, or want a lens that helps you identify colors in the traffic lights, your eye doctor can offer various options, including some excellent photochromic glasses that are now available. Also ask about anti-reflective coating. The anti-reflective coating helps cut down on glare and actually increases the amount of light getting to the eye by about 8 percent. The additional light is especially important if you have difficulty with contrast. Some of these lenses smudge easily, and many patients have trouble cleaning them. It isn't difficult to do with soap and water or an alcohol solution, but it does take extra effort.

If You Are Still Driving at Night

All drivers are disadvantaged when driving at night. Instead of the normal visual field of 180 degrees, the range is reduced to approximately 40 degrees—the distance exposed by your headlights. Visual acuity is also reduced because of a reduction in the contrast of objects seen. These elements make driving at night difficult for almost everyone. When combined with the slower reaction time of an older driver and a loss of vision from AMD, they are particularly problematic.

You always want to give your eyes time to adjust to the darkness. Your eyes have the same difficulty when you leave a brightly lit home to go out and get into a car in the evening as they do when you enter a darkened movie theater. Get into the car and sit for a few minutes before attempting to drive. Also, if you will be driving to or from a new neighborhood at night, you should consider taking a trial run during the day.

Though you will occasionally see ads for "night driving glasses," the claims being made are bogus. The only lenses that can be safely worn at night while driving are clear lenses or lenses with anti-reflective coating. Tinted glasses should never be worn for driving at night.

The glare from halogen headlights, especially from high-mounted vehicles such as sports utility vehicles, can seriously impair a person's visual acuity for as long as twenty to thirty minutes. In addition to the anti-reflective coating on your glasses, another strategy to reduce glare from headlights is to try looking slightly to the left or to the right of oncoming headlights.

Some new models of cars are being outfitted with infrared technology (first used by the military during Desert Storm) that permits night drivers to see objects that are beyond the normal field of vision revealed by headlights. The system works by sending out an infrared beam that is not visible to oncoming cars; the information gathered is then displayed in a low spot on the windshield where it doesn't impede your view for driving. However, those with AMD may find that the beam adds glare to the windshield or that the infrared reflection is bothersome when it is reflected on the windshield. As the adaptation of the technology for passenger cars is improved, it will be easier to judge how helpful it will be for those with AMD.

Making the decision not to drive at night should be one of the first restrictions you place on yourself. Whether we have AMD or not, studies show that by age sixty our night vision is significantly worse and it becomes harder to see objects that aren't moving.

Ensuring Optimum Conditions

Precautions can be taken in other areas as well. Stay off the road during bad weather, rush hour, and any period of the day that makes it more difficult for you to see. Early morning sun and sunset may create too much glare; gray winter afternoons may reduce contrast. Once you know when your bad times are, you can schedule errands and appointments so that you needn't be on the road at those times.

If you carry a cellular telephone, turn it off while driving or resolve that you won't answer it. If you need to place an outgoing call, pull off the road into a safe place where you can be easily seen by other drivers. Start and complete your call while at a full stop. Other distractions of this sort include smoking or drinking coffee or sodas while driving.

While the radio news can be helpful for weather and traffic updates, consider turning it down or off when you are in a lot of traffic. The radio can be distracting, and may reduce your ability to hear important traffic sounds around you.

If you have grandchildren with you, make sure they are in car seats, or in the backseat if they are too old for a car seat, and always in a restraint system. It goes without saying that you should wear your own seat belt at all times.

If you travel with a pet—even just to the vet—consider crating the animal, or putting it in one of the new dog restraint systems. No driver should have to cope with an animal moving around unexpectedly.

Safe Driving Techniques

Plan your route in advance, and select one that will be less heavily traveled and less demanding. (You can do this easily by visiting one of the Internet map sites.) Avoid intersections without signals, and think about whether or not you'll have to make a left turn without a left turn arrow. For that matter, you should follow all driving regulations for signaling your intentions to turn or to change lanes.

As you drive, you should constantly be scanning and observing three elements:

1. characteristics of the road (straight, curving, two- or four-lane, etc.)
2. traffic control devices, taking particular care at uncontrolled intersections
3. other road users—both other cars as well as pedestrians, who deserve utmost caution

Check your mirrors frequently. And if you are still driving at night, remember about the day/night settings. The proper setting can help reduce glare.

One useful step is to drive with your low beams (not parking lights) on both day and night. In Canada all cars now must have "daytime running lights," lights that are turned on whenever the car is running. This requirement is under consideration in the United States as well. Write to your representative about making this a law. Both drivers and pedestrians with AMD report that they can see cars in the daytime much better if the car's lights are on. By observing this practice, you will heighten the visibility of the car you are driving, and you may successfully remind other drivers of this safe practice, too.

Drive with a wide area of safety in front of you; a three-second safety cushion is recommended. To determine this, find a stationary object—a tree or a traffic post—along the side of the road. Once the car ahead of you passes it, you should be able to count "1001, 1002, 1003" before arriving at the same object. Driving too closely reduces the time you have to react to what is happening ahead of you.

Good Driving Isn't in the Eyes Alone

Ninety percent of the sensory information required for driving is visual. However, you can use your other senses and physical abilities to heighten traffic awareness to some extent.

The ability to react is helpful if you exercise regularly and stay in good physical condition. Good blood flow and enough flexibility to turn your head and shoulders all the way to the left and right to check the road are all vital to good driving.

Have your hearing checked regularly. Traffic sounds, sirens, and the toots of car horns are all important signals to drivers about what is happening on the road. Taking in sensory information of other types will supplement your eyesight. Sirens often seem to come out of nowhere, and you'll be forewarned of accidents or other tie-ups if you hear horns up ahead or screeching tires.

To compensate for slower reaction time, some drivers drive more slowly. This can be a hazard on the highway, but it is usually an acceptable alternative when driving on local roads.

Social drinking and driving should be avoided. If you attend a party or go out for a meal and would like to have a drink, ask someone else to drive you home or plan to take a taxi. After age fifty-five, our bodies metabolize food and drink, including alcohol, more slowly. The alcohol stays in the body longer, prolonging the effect it has on judgment and response time. In addition, the U.S. Food and Drug Administration reports that 50 percent of all medications taken by older people interact poorly with alcohol, further increasing your risk of not being fully alert.

If you are going to a new destination and someone is in the car with you, enlist their help with reading maps and checking street signs. This permits you to keep your focus on the road.

Avoiding Accidents

According to the AARP, older drivers commonly make two mistakes. The first is the failure to yield the right of way. This dangerous practice isn't because older people feel they "own the road," but more likely because they fail to see another car that has the right of way. As a driver, you need to become a more active "looker," moving your head more to be certain that you're taking in the complete scene around you. If you have a passenger, you might enlist help.

The second common mistake is making improper left turns. Left turns across a busy street or several lanes of traffic can be harrowing if there's no green arrow to provide time for a protected turn. The AARP recommends a cautious cure for this one: Avoid the left turn altogether by making three right turns (going around the block) when practical. This method is an excellent solution when streets are laid out in a grid pattern. When they aren't, and the oncoming traffic is very heavy, your next best alternative is to continue along the street until you find a light with a left turn signal. Make the left and then find a spot to turn around and come back to the store or the street that is your destination.

On an Internet site dedicated to low-vision driving, one person with a restricted license posted the following:

"Driving is not a right. It is a privilege, regardless of your vision . . . [Once you've been diagnosed with an eye condition], you can never become 100 percent dependent on the fact that you are licensed to drive. There will be times when you won't be able to (snow, ice, heavy rain or fog, very bright sun, etc.) and it is important not to do so. You can still get to work or do errands. Take the bus, call a cab, walk, or bike. You can still get around. Trust me. I've been there."

When to Stop Driving

One need only talk to former drivers who have had to stop driving for all types of reasons, ranging from blackout episodes to frailty, to know that giving up the freedom gained by driving a car is a tremendous loss. People often feel isolated and resent not being able to get into the car to run a quick errand or to meet someone for lunch without having to plan ahead how to get there.

Some people with AMD say "you just know" when it's time to quit. One woman told how she left her house, drove a few blocks, and then went right back home, knowing she never wanted to get behind the wheel again.

Many resist for as long as possible. One woman finally made the decision, which her children had been nagging her to make, when she made a right turn into traffic just in front of a gray-colored truck. There was little contrast between the truck and the gray sky, and she simply didn't see it. Others are corraled by family members who finally "take away the keys." And some linger on until their doctor pronounces them unfit to drive, or they can no longer pass the driving test.

If you have gradually been cutting back on your driving by not driving at night or using buses or taxis when the weather is bad, this change may not be as unsettling as it is for someone who must make the decision suddenly. If you realize there are options, the transition is much easier.

Some people move once they realize they will be unable to drive. One woman gave up her home and took an apartment in New York City, where public transportation is easily available. A Midwesterner selected a home that was within walking distance of a grocery store as well as near a bus stop with two bus lines. Obviously, moving must fit with your overall needs in life, but if you are considering a move anyway, keep in mind your new requirements for public transportation and services to which you can walk easily.

The inability to drive puts into motion a set of challenging decisions that need to be made. Give yourself time. Deciding on your own that it's time to quit is probably the least painful way to come to terms with this issue. In the coming months and years it will be important to review your driving skills regularly:

- Have you been in an accident recently?
- Do people frequently honk at you? Not a good sign.
- Do you become flustered more often than not when driving?
- Do you find driving exhausting?
- Is sunlight growing more problematic? Before factoring this in, consult with your optometrist and make certain you have glasses that cut glare and heighten contrast (see Chapter 7).

If your answers to the above questions are in the "sort of" range, you still have a few alternatives. Using driving simulation tests, a study was conducted with people who had AMD. They performed poorly, yet their accident rate was excellent. Why? They seem to have self-regulated themselves, driving enough to remain independent, but not in areas or at times that put them in jeopardy. Almost none drove at night, and the driving they did was on back roads at off-hours.

So consider what restrictions you can place on yourself that will let you do errands or get to work without driving in the worst traffic.

When you consider optimum times of day, don't ever forget the child with the ball. A fully sighted driver is hard-pressed to react quickly if a child dashes out into the street. So do what you can to avoid streets with many children, or times of day when children tend to be playing in the front yard.

Making Other Arrangements

Even before you reach the point when you think it's better not to drive, begin to research your alternatives. If you investigate these services now, you'll find the transition will be easier, and you'll feel in control again. What's more, you may find that a combination works. For instance, you might drive yourself on back roads to do some errands in the morning. Later in the day you might get to the class you're taking or the concert that night by taking the bus or calling a cab. You'll soon find you can continue to do all the things you used to do. You may have to allow a little more time, but you'll be freed of the responsibility and the worry.

You should also consider the alternatives available in your community. Some towns have transportation provisions for seniors. It may be a shuttle bus that comes when you call it, or a network of volunteers that serve as pseudo-cabbies for those who need drivers. You may pay by the ride only, or there may be a membership fee with a lower per-ride fee.

Many churches and temples have a regular network of volunteers who are willing to provide transportation to and from events. Availing yourself of this option may lead you to other volunteer networks.

In major cities like New York, Washington, Boston, and San Francisco, public transportation is commonly used by everyone, and you'll find that routinely navigating the city by subway and bus becomes second nature. Elsewhere, use of public transportation may not be widespread, but don't be put off by your sighted friends who denigrate public transportation with comments like "The bus depot looks so dirty" (Have they been in it recently? Do they *know* it's dirty?) or "I'd be nervous riding buses. You never know who might sit next to you." Those who have taken the leap report that people watching on buses can be first-rate. You do take a little longer to get around by public transportation, but are you really in such a rush?

To learn what options are available in your area, contact the transit agency or your local office on aging. These organizations have lists of what is available. If you find no appropriate local listing, look under state government listings; the appropriate state agency will tell you whom to call in your area.

Ask your library to order *Finding Wheels: A Curriculum for Nondrivers with Visual Impairments for Gaining Control of Transportation Needs* (January 2000, Pro Ed, Austin, Texas) by Anne Lesley Corn and L. Penny Rosenblum. Though the book is written to inspire visually impaired teens to find other ways to get around, both authors are visually impaired, and their advice can be applied to adults as well.

Using Public Transportation

Here are some tips that will help. First, if you have to cross a street to get to the bus stop or to a subway station, do so carefully. Cross at a light, ask someone for help, or use the skills taught you by an orientation and mobility specialist to know when it's safe to cross. Likewise, if you can't read the bus or subway numbers, ask someone to identify the bus or subway.

Stock up on coins or on tokens if your community uses them. (Ask about discounts.) You can slip one into your pocket so you needn't find it in your wallet once the bus comes.

At a train station or a subway platform, stand away from the edge of the platform, preferably near a pillar or stairway.

This will keep you out of danger of being jostled too close to the edge.

One of the great benefits of public transportation is that it frees you to do other things. Instead of focusing on the road, you can observe people around you (a frequently fascinating activity) or listen to a book. Purchase, or put on your wish list, a cassette player with an earpiece. Now you can take an audio book along with you. That way the time you're on the bus, train, or subway will fly by.

Taxis or Contract Drivers

Calling a cab regularly or using a part-time driver with whom you've made some type of contractual (verbal or written) agreement may seem like an extravagance, but before you cross it off as an option, consider this. If you own a car, pay for insurance, and spend money on gas, upkeep, and parking, that's quite a big expense each year. Estimate what your annual costs are for your automobile and divide that figure by fifty-two weeks. This gives you the amount per week you could easily spend on transportation when you no longer have the expense of owning and maintaining a car.

Some communities offer discount coupons for taxi service to senior citizens or those with disabilities. Ask if any sort of discount is available in your area.

While you will probably rely on friends and family for some of your transportation needs, you can certainly afford to take a few cabs or even hire a driver for several afternoons per week. Hiring a retired person or a college student to do some driving for you offers the advantage of privacy. Many people feel much more comfortable knowing the person who will be picking them up.

To find someone, run an ad for a "part-time driver." A good number of retired people have no desire to work full-time, but they would like some extra spending money. Many college students are more than willing to drive you to a meeting and do homework until the meeting is concluded and you're ready to be driven home. Negotiate a per-ride or per-hour rate that is agreeable to both parties, and you've created another way to get around. One woman kept her car to be used by the college student she hired. Rather than paying in cash, she permitted the student to use the car for part of the week as the student's "salary" for specified driving hours. Both were delighted with the arrangement.

When You Must Leave the Driving to Others

Without doubt, learning to rely on others for transportation requires an adjustment. Here are some suggestions on making it work out satisfactorily to all:

Plan ahead. Driving offers flexibility. You can hop into the car and run out for groceries, and if you forget something, you can always go back out again. Now you'll need to be organized. If you haven't already been doing so, start keeping detailed lists. Don't leave anything to memory. When you do go out, you'll know exactly where you need to go and what you need to buy.

Allow extra time. Whether waiting for a bus or a cab or getting a ride with a friend, you will find that other forms of transportation are not as efficient as driving your own car.

Be independent at least some of the time. You may have a spouse who is still driving or children who live in the area. Be grateful for their availability, and then continue to explore other ways to get around such as buses or cabs. Sure, a spouse, son, or daughter who will go with you to a concert or come along to a doctor's appointment with you is very helpful. Yet you will feel better if you make your own plans, and you'll lessen any possible strain that overdependence might place on a relationship.

Friends will be happy to help, but use them wisely. If a friend is going to the store anyway, hop a ride—you'll both have a better time. In general, friends probably won't mind driving you on errands when they are going out anyway. However, try to avoid using them as a regular taxi service. People will no doubt most enjoy joining you for excursions such as picking out a gift for someone, or selecting some new clothing, when you want the opinion of a friend. Almost anyone would be happy to give you a lift to a concert or a town meeting.

Find creative ways to repay favors. If you ride frequently with a friend, offer to buy the next tank of gas, or purchase a little gift, bake something, or pay for dinner, a concert, or the movies. Even your spouse deserves a special acknowledgment.

Before ending the chapter, let's take a glimpse into the future. In the next few years new technology will benefit those with AMD and may extend the driving days of low-vision drivers. In addition to the infrared technology being added to cars to make night driving easier, the global positioning satellites that are being installed in some vehicles will make navigating easier. After entering an address into a computer that receives the satellite signal, drivers will receive verbal instructions as to how to proceed, complete with exact information on where to turn and how far to travel between landmarks. Such improvements will let drivers concentrate on driving with less to worry about—providing a longer driving life.

13

Out and About

Getting out of the house and among people is a great mood lifter. If you work or have a steady volunteer commitment, then you already understand the benefits of maintaining contact with the world around you. For those who have recently retired or moved—or for those tempted to withdraw from life because of difficulty seeing—we urge you to get proper training from an orientation and mobility specialist who can help assure safe navigation, use the information in this chapter, and stay active and involved.

For many people with macular degeneration, peripheral vision can remain quite strong for a long time. While doing close work or seeing faces may become more difficult, most people still see well enough to do what they want.

The man in his late seventies who still travels the world, the innumerable people who continue to go to work each day, the doctor who continues to play tennis (albeit a slower game), and the woman who still plays golf—all prove that people with AMD continue to lead active and busy lives.

Consider the woman in her eighties who recently arrived by subway for her appointment at the New York Lighthouse:

"You came by subway?" her eye-care professional asked.

"Oh, yes. It was the fastest way to get here after my dance class," she replied.

General Mobility

Fully sighted people enjoy the luxury of seeing far more than is necessary. It is, indeed, very convenient and interesting to be able to see a full panorama of the world around you when you are walking, but you do not *need* that much information in order to make your way down the street.

Safe navigation by foot requires a general awareness of the environment as well as up-to-date information on the space immediately in front of you to avoid any obstacles. Learning other ways to absorb information provides you with the necessary skills to travel safely on your own.

Getting around is an important safety issue, and for that reason, it is important to get help with this training from an orientation and mobility specialist. (Contact a vision-rehabilitation center in your area or your state's agency for the vision impaired.)

Use the Vision You Have

Scanning what's ahead is the best way to take in meaningful information as you walk. By letting your eyes traverse the territory systematically, you'll get a more complete picture than if your eyes dart here and there.

Tracing a natural line with your eyes will provide you with directional information. Even if your central vision is quite poor, your peripheral vision will show you the line where the grass and the sidewalk meet or, in a city, the line of the buildings. When you reach a corner or a "junction," you'll know a new decision must be made as to which way to turn.

Tracking anything with a predictable pattern of movement can provide you with temporary guidance. For example, on a busy city street you can follow a person ahead of you. When he steps down, you know that a curb is coming up.

Spotting stationary landmarks is helpful in orienting yourself. Once you reach the statue, you know it's time to turn left, for example. Or spotting the bottom of a traffic signal pole can also lead you to trace the pole to the top, where you can use your peripheral vision to see the light.

Rely More on Your Hearing

When we were children we learned to "Stop, look, and listen" before we crossed the street. Now that the "looking" part of this instructional message is less reliable, it is time to gather more information with your ears.

The whereabouts of cars, emergency equipment with sirens, and people nearby can all be absorbed by listening, as can the change of the light signals or the fact that you have gone past a large building. Yes, it is possible to "hear" the end of a building: In cities like New York, one of the ways to identify your whereabouts is to "listen" to the building; because it naturally blocks and reflects sound, the full sounds of the street will only be heard once you go beyond it. You may also notice changes like a different wind flow on your face, or the sun suddenly breaking through to warm you. As you become more experienced, these are additional tools to use in identifying street corners.

An orientation and mobility specialist can help sensitize you to what and how to listen in your community.

Additional Hints for Navigating the Streets

It's best to decide your jaywalking days are over. If your central vision has deteriorated to the point that a car can "come out of nowhere," you should cross at street corners and follow the traffic lights.

Don't hesitate to ask for help at a street corner. Most people like being helpful because they hope a stranger will do the same for someone they love.

Making Streets More Accessible

Some communities are installing what are called accessible pedestrian signals (APS). These provide "walk/don't walk" information for the visually impaired by using audible tones, verbal messages, and/or tactile vibrating devices. Some signals automatically emit a beep, a click, or a birdcall of sorts; others are designed so that a button must be pressed to get the sound. These buttons give off "locator" tones, so the person wishing to cross a street can find where to activate the signal.

Though all these systems are well intended, those with visual impairments indicate that some designs are better than others. For example, the style that emits a continuous beeping can actually be dangerous if it masks regular traffic sounds—an important part of crossing the street to a person with reduced vision. To explore how to bring accessible pedestrian signals to your community, contact Lighthouse International for more information.

In some cities—San Francisco, for one—experimental systems are showing the way of the future. Equipped with a handheld receiver, a visually impaired person can enter an area that has been equipped to give signals. By clicking his receiver, he can hear a voice message about the status of the crosswalk signal, the name of the cross street, and even the number of traffic lanes that must be crossed.

If someone is walking with you to assist you, grip the person's arm just above the elbow—the other person shouldn't take your arm. Your "guide" should walk about a half pace ahead of you, so that you can feel and follow his or her movements. It is also helpful if this person warns you of what's coming up (a turn, a stop, a door).

If you are guided into a building or if the lighting is bad outdoors, ask to be led to a wall or to the information desk. This will provide you with a way of getting oriented; being left in the middle of an open space can be frightening.

The White Cane and the Guide Dog

Many of you will never need this type of help; others may find that additional aid would be welcome some or all of the time. By contacting your state's Commission for the Blind, or asking at a vision-rehabilitation center near you, you can locate an orientation and mobility training specialist who can help you identify whether either a cane or a dog would be helpful in your circumstances. These professionals can also provide you with proper training in the use of the cane. If the orientation and mobility specialist feels you are a good candidate for a guide dog, he or she will help you locate a guide-dog school, where you will receive specialized training in using a dog.

White Cane

If you find that your vision is not always adequate for navigation or for identifying obstacles, a white cane is a logical choice. The cane offers navigational help and is a legally recognized signal to others that you may not see them. Canes are available in a collapsible style, so if you navigate on your own to an appointment in the afternoon, when you leave at dusk, you can use the cane you've carried in a purse or briefcase. An orientation and mobility specialist will work with you to help you use the cane safely.

Guide Dog

Although some people with AMD do get guide dogs, experts point out that a dog is best used by a person who sees very little or not at all. Because most people with macular degeneration retain a good amount of peripheral vision, a guide dog is usually not a first option. To maintain good habits, the dog needs to be fully in charge at all times that he is working. It is confusing for the dog if a person sometimes gets himself around an obstacle and sometimes expects the dog to do it.

Special training is necessary for using a cane or for working with a guide dog. An orientation and mobility specialist can help with both.

Getting Where You Need To and Getting Things Done

Using the navigation systems just described, you will gain confidence and skill as you continue to be out and about. To provide even more help, you'll find there are a few tools that come in handy. The first is the telescopic aid described in Chapter 8. Identifying street signs and building addresses takes a little longer using this device, but at least it will permit you to read signs when necessary.

A pocket flashlight is also a good item to have handy. Being able to illuminate a building directory, an elevator number, or a price tag on a possible purchase will provide you with a greater feeling of control.

A magnifier, ideally one you wear on a chain around your neck, also comes in handy. The hard-to-read price tag, store label, or restaurant receipt may now be accessible to you if you have both a magnifier and a flashlight.

Public Spaces

Once you go in after being outside, take a few moments to let your eyes adjust. Older people—and those with AMD in particular—often find that it takes them longer to recover their sight when switching from a bright environment to a dim one.

Restaurants and theaters can be very difficult to navigate because of the dim lighting. Rather than avoid these places or resent the fact that they are so dark, use your pocket flashlight when you need to. It may help in reading a menu or getting to the bathroom.

Elevators tend to be dimly lit, and seeing the numbers on the buttons can be hard. Though some elevators have raised numbers, for the most part your best source of help will be someone on the elevator with you. If you're alone, bend down so that your eyes are close to the panel, and use your pocket flashlight. Modern elevators beep as each floor is passed. By paying attention, you'll know when it's time to get off.

Shopping for Groceries

Having a complete list and shopping consistently at one store can make grocery shopping easier. To have a good shopping list week after week, start by creating a master list for your particular store. Visit the store once to identify the whereabouts of the different products, and write down the categories of food based on your store's floor plan, starting in the aisle where you normally begin anyway. If produce is in Aisle 1 and baked goods are in Aisle 2, then these items would go first on your list. After walking through the store, you might have a list that looks like this:

GROCERY LIST

Fruits and Vegetables	Baked Goods	Drinks
Household Cleaning Items	Paper Goods	Staples/ Seasonings
Canned Goods	Meats and Fish	Dairy
Frozen Foods	Miscellaneous	

If you need to print using very large letters, use more than one page for your list, leaving additional space between categories. Then make fifteen to twenty photocopies of the list. If yours is more than one page, staple the pages together. Each week you will start fresh with a new list on which to write what you need.

You can remove labels from the jars, cans, or boxes of your favorite brands. Sometimes matching labels is easier than reading them, particularly when companies use fancy cursive writing to identify their product. An excellent place to store these labels is in a "coupon billfold," a special wallet or holder for coupons.

If you need only a few things and don't want to bother with a written list, perhaps you should use one of the digital recorders (described in Chapter 8). A good recorder has several different "files" for reminders, and you can dedicate one to groceries. After recording the items as you think of them, take the recorder with you and use it as an audio reminder of what you need to buy. This is a cumbersome way to shop for a large number of groceries, but it's an excellent way to remind yourself of six or seven items. Once you've completed the list, you can simply reuse the file to record another short list of items.

Many people have trouble with glare from the overhead fluorescent store lights. Try wearing a visor or a baseball cap when you shop. You'll be surprised at how reducing the glare helps you see.

Touch and smell can help you choose fresh fruits and vegetables. You already know how to differentiate an apple from a pear, to feel for soft spots, check the weight, and smell the sweetness. If certain items come pre-bagged, such as grapes, you may want to check with another shopper.

If your vision is such that even these solutions leave you struggling to identify the various canned good labels or the cuts of meat and their prices, talk to your store manager. Most stores will provide someone to go through the aisles with you to help select your purchases.

Most people like to select their own meat and fresh fruit and vegetables. However, certain items—for example, paper goods, drinks, bulky items—can be ordered by phone or computer and delivered. Delivery services exist in major cities, or if you're on the Internet, you may find that one of the online grocery companies services your area. In many cases you can leave a standing order, and the basics will be sent to you each week.

Shopping for Clothes

If you shop at smaller stores, you will get to know the staff. The small boutique nearby may not have the selection a department store does, but a good store owner will help you find clothing that works for you and may even call you when they get in something that would be "perfect."

If you have a magnifier and/or flashlight, you can use them to read prices and clothing care labels. For colors that are difficult to identify, shop with a friend who can advise you.

Social Contact

When you have macular degeneration, social situations can sometimes put you at a disadvantage. You look the same as you always did, and certain things you do, such as walking into a room unaided, or picking up something from the floor, may indicate to others that you see just fine. What others can't be expected to understand is that you may not recognize faces. As a result, you may not pick out a friend in a group, and you may be puzzled when that person comes up and greets you warmly.

Some people with AMD respond by withdrawing from social situations. Although this may protect a person from some social awkwardness, such isolation creates all sorts of other difficulties. Being alone is a major contributor to depression. Having contact with other people, despite a few uneasy moments, is absolutely vital to coping with macular degeneration.

Recognizing that social situations present specific challenges provides the opportunity to strategize. If you're attending an event with a spouse or friend, ask her to identify by name the people who approach the two of you. If you're attending alone, or if you and your friend/spouse separate for part of the evening, you have two choices. When Bill meets someone, he openly requests, "Come closer. I can't see your face." Terry simply enjoys being with people and talks to whomever she comes across at a party. "I may eventually figure out who they are based on their voice or from a comment they make, but I often leave a party having no idea who some of the people were—but that's okay. I have a good time," she says. "I used to run a store, so I'm accustomed to talking to strangers, and I've always enjoyed it."

Introduce yourself with confidence, and smile as the conversation merits it. As you talk, turn toward the person who is speaking. In turn, they'll talk directly to you. Remember, unlike other types of disabilities, you don't look any different—the person has no reason to suspect you don't see him fully.

If the person expresses surprise that you don't recognize her, use it as an opportunity to briefly explain your vision loss. While you don't want to become someone who buttonholes people and lectures them about getting their eyes examined, not that many people know about AMD. If you educate others about your experience, it may inspire them to be more watchful for themselves or their family members. Many people have become accustomed to explaining: "I have low vision (or macular degeneration), and because I don't have much central vision, I can't identify who you are."

People often report difficulty hearing people as their vision dims, partly because they've relied on facial expression and lip movements to help them grasp meaning. You may find you need to get used to listening carefully, or if you are concerned, get your hearing checked. The use of hearing aids has grown rapidly, and being fit for one is relatively simple and very helpful.

You can also use the trick of concentrating on voices and identifying characteristics of friends and family. One cousin may have a habit of clearing his throat; an aunt may play with her chain necklace. As you rely less on your ability to see facial features, see what other characteristics you can identify. As you become an expert listener, you may be surprised by how much of a person's mood is conveyed by voice alone. For example, a chipper voice will almost certainly come from a person with a smile.

Maintain a sense of humor. From going into the wrong bathroom to striking up a conversation with a stranger, you'll probably have your fair share of mishaps. Rather than feeling self-conscious, try to let yourself enjoy a good laugh.

Ways to Stay Active

If there's something you'd like to do but can't figure out how to accomplish, pose the question to your low-vision specialist. Chances are excellent that he will find a way—or refer you to someone who can. Before starting an exercise program, check with both your eye doctor and your regular doctor first.

Getting Regular Exercise

If you enjoy walking or running, think about where you can do it safely. If you have a school track near your home, walk there to exercise. Then you won't have to worry about traffic. Otherwise, try to develop a route that does not involve crossing streets. Some people use a park. Exercising with a friend will help you maintain discipline, and it also provides additional safety. Others meet with friends at a mall and walk before the serious shoppers arrive.

Wearing identification is important for anyone who exercises outside the home. Put a label in something that you always carry with you.

A regular walking stick may give you a feeling of security, particularly if you walk in an area where the terrain isn't even.

Take an exercise class. Today there are classes in so many disciplines, it is hard not to find something you would like. Tai chi and yoga are both wonderful methods of putting your muscles to work, and aerobic classes can also be a lot of fun. What's more, you benefit in two ways: You'll get your exercise and spend some time with people as well. A scheduled exercise class is also a great way to make sure you get out of the house regularly.

Exercising to a video offers control over when you exercise as well as the comfort of being in your own home. Isometric exercises, the systematic tightening and relaxing of your muscles, can also be done safely at convenient moments throughout the day. Or, if you have access to an indoor pool, swimming is an excellent form of regular exercise.

Sports

You may believe your days on the tennis court are over, but think again. One doctor with macular degeneration can no longer play the high-speed tennis he once enjoyed, but he has found several partners with whom to play a more relaxed game. "While I originally slowed down because of my eyes, to tell you the truth, my knees wouldn't have held out much longer for my old style of play anyway," he notes. "I still really enjoy the game."

Golf is another sport that people with AMD still play with enthusiasm. One woman points out that you often must rely on your partner to spot your ball, and some partners prove to be better than others. "People always invite me to go out with them, but I'm choosy as to whom I play with. I need someone who will reliably remember to tell me where I've hit the ball," she says. "Even when they mean well, people sometimes forget about it after the first hole or two." Once they get to the putting green, she reports that though her vision loss is quite severe, she still has enough peripheral vision that she's quite good at completing the hole. "I love to play. It gets me outdoors, and I'm still doing something I love."

Check with your low-vision specialist about any sport you choose to pursue. She may have suggestions about adaptive devices or special techniques that will help. Here are some ideas to keep in mind:

- Shatterproof glasses that block the sunlight and reduce glare are invaluable for outdoor sports.
- In some sports, a handheld telescope may be helpful. Some golfers use it before their first shot to locate the hole.
- Contrast is always helpful. Golf balls, tennis balls, skis, and fishing lures come in fluorescent colors, making them

easier to see. In golf, your partner can also help you create contrast. Ask him to frame the hole with his shoes
(stand with his feet forming a right angle) to provide
contrast to help you make your best shot.

- In tennis, the size of the racquet can make a difference.
  Select one with a large sweet spot.
- Adaptive devices make some sports easier to play.
  There are now bowling guide rails to improve bowling
  games, and lap swimmers can use the flotation lane
  dividers.

As for spectator sports, you can still enjoy going along
with friends or family to baseball, football, and basketball
games. Baseball, with the crack of the bat and the roar of the
crowd, is particularly fun because the game's pattern is predictable. Take along a transistor radio with an earpiece (you
may have always done this anyway). Between the reporting by
the announcers, the smells and sounds of attending a sporting
event, and the camaraderie of sharing an activity with other
people, you're guaranteed a good outing.

Cultural Activities

Countless people with AMD attend the theater. Many use
regular binoculars for better viewing, but other devices can
also be prescribed that make seeing the stage easier. In addition, some theaters provide headsets with auditory descriptions of the visual performances.

Museums and art galleries sometimes offer programs in
large print or on cassette, and many offer auditory guided
tours with enhanced descriptions of displays. New Yorkers say
that the tours at the Metropolitan Museum of Art are first-

rate. Call your local museums and ask what is available. Still other galleries are beginning to offer "hands-on" exhibits for adults where the art can be explored by touch.

Hobbies

Tell your low-vision specialist what your hobbies are and find out what aids and devices are available. If you enjoy a good card game, for example, ask about what visual aids might be helpful. Certain types of bifocals allow you to see the cards in your hand as well as those on the table. Specially designed telescopic prescriptive lenses are also available, so see if you're a candidate for these or maybe for a special head-mounted electronic system. In addition, try the following:

- Use large-print playing cards, available through specialty stores.
- Play cards on contrasting surfaces.
- Take along a gooseneck lamp to make viewing the cards easier.

As for gardening, you might want to use large-print markers to label what you're growing. For contrast, you can paint tools or tool handles. That way if you put down a trowel, you'll be able to find it again. Painting the blade of a hoe white will provide better contrast with the ground.

Volunteer Work

Volunteering offers many benefits. Dedicating yourself to a cause or a particular project puts you in contact with people and offers exercise for the mind, heart, and soul. People with AMD take on service projects ranging from town committees to nonprofit boards. They do work that is needed, they have something different to think about, and many find it easier to accept help from others when they are giving back.

Finding volunteer work when you have AMD is no different from before. Ask friends, call organizations that are of interest to you, and go through the local newspaper. Of course, the amount of time required and where meetings are held, or where the volunteer work is performed, will be deciding factors—just as they were before.

If you're so motivated, your current experience is a source for a wide range of ideas. Look around your own community and think about how people with low vision could be better served. Perhaps you could offer to implement a program at the library where volunteers would be available to read to people with low vision. Funds could be raised for a reading machine. Would you like to start a campaign for better signs or for bringing accessible pedestrian signals to your community? Or why not gather friends to write letters to Congress and to car manufacturers about making daytime running lights a requirement on future cars? Imagine what would happen in your community if you convinced the local government to create contrast at corner curbs, using nothing fancier than a bucket of paint. Or organize a meeting of local architects and explain to them what design modifications would help people with macular degeneration get around more easily. One simple element among the many used at the Lighthouse is painting doorways in a color that contrasts with the color of the walls. That very simple change can make a great deal of difference to someone with AMD.

Think of what interests you most—you could really make a difference.

Your world does not have to close in just because you don't see it as well. Whether you're walking, going out with friends, or helping others, you are the one who determines how much of life you want to enjoy. So get trained, get out, get about, and stay involved.

14

Advice for Others

People mean well, but in their attempts to help you, they often unintentionally do anything but. The next time someone grabs your arm to help you get somewhere or shouts at you because they think difficulty seeing also means difficulty hearing, you'll begin to realize that *they* need a handbook about macular degeneration almost as much as you do.

In all likelihood, you've shared with those close to you some of the information in this book, and you've told them what is known about various treatments. Now it's time to let them know a little more. If they read the following short chapter themselves, they will learn how best to act on their very admirable intentions.

The first thing your friends and family should know is that they must resist being overprotective. While you may need them to help you locate the rehabilitation services in your area, they should be aware that the goal is for you to learn to do as much as you can for yourself. While the tendency to be overprotective is natural, neither you nor they will benefit if you come to rely on them for things you are capable of doing for yourself.

If necessary, invite friends or family to come to one of your sessions with a vision-rehabilitation therapist or an orientation and mobility specialist. They will feel reassured by seeing how much you can expect to do on your own.

Coping with Depression

Experts say that a person's basic personality tends to determine how they handle adversity. The person who has always met difficulties head on is likely to manage macular degeneration in the same way. Those who have always resisted change are likely to do so now. However, sometimes people rise to the challenge. After worrying for years about all the bad things that could happen, they finally gain the strength to cope, when something really bad does happen.

"My father is in denial that anything is wrong," says Karen. "When he visits my house and watches any television, he stands right by the television and looks at it from the side. His doctor has told him what he has, but every time we suggest taking him for a low-vision evaluation, he is very resistant."

"Denial can be a common defense against depression," says Amy Horowitz, senior vice president for research and evaluation for Lighthouse International, where she has overseen studies on depression and vision loss. "Particularly for the person who is diagnosed early and is not yet having much functional vision loss, it is a protective strategy. The person fears going blind, and the thought is too much of an assault."

Both denial and depression are normal at the beginning, but they become unhealthy if the emotional state continues past the time when a person starts to need additional help. The earlier a person begins to explore his options and learn about adaptive techniques, the easier time he will have adjusting to the changes in vision. So it's important to look for professional help if the depression goes on too long.

If you are concerned that your friend or loved one has become depressed, you should watch for the following signs:

- has been "down" for many weeks
- stays in bed and has little interest in what is going on
- is tearful, weepy, or sad
- takes diminished pleasure in outings or seeing the grandchildren, or something that used to lift the spirits
- gives up things that don't require strong vision (the person who no longer listens to their favorite radio program may be clinically depressed)
- experiences changes in sleep patterns, either sleeping too much or not enough
- has a significant weight change in either direction
- takes pleasure in very few activities
- seems to change baseline personality
- has a major change in energy level, either seeming too restless or lethargic
- has difficulty concentrating
- is preoccupied with the disease, to the point that it is her sole focus, without being able to take steps to improve her situation
- indicates that he isn't worth anyone going to any trouble for
- makes comments about death or suicide
- refuses treatment

If a person exhibits any of these signs for several weeks or more, seek help for her. Some vision-rehabilitation centers have mental health professionals on staff, or a good internist or gerontologist may offer recommendations. If therapy is needed, some professionals work with people on a sliding scale. The National Association of Family Services is one place to contact for additional help. Depression can be treated, and if the person starts feeling better, it may motivate her to tackle new challenges associated with learning to live with macular degeneration.

Friends and family members often help the most by listening. "Ask how he or she is feeling," recommends psychologist Dr. Lisa Weiss. "Some people want to talk about it; some people don't, but by asking directly, you'll get a sense of their level of acceptance. One person may immediately launch into their emotional reaction; others may still be trying to come to terms with what may lie ahead."

"I started sending my mother articles and clippings about macular degeneration after she told me she had it," says Yolanda. "At the time, her vision was still quite good, and I think she was taking time to adjust to the news. Sending her newspaper clippings about driving with bioptic glasses when she was still perfectly capable of driving normally probably just depressed her more. I should have asked her more about what she was experiencing instead of pushing ahead to try to find solutions for problems that hadn't even occurred."

Living with Someone Who Has Low Vision

First off, ask what would be helpful. He may have specific tasks that are difficult to do yet handles the rest of them the same as always. You may find that the one thing the person hates is dealing with the grocery store because of the glare. If the two of you go together, the process may become much easier.

If the person turns you down, offer help again later on. Too often offers of help dwindle as time goes on, and if you remain available, the other person may come around.

Find out whether there is a time of day that is particularly difficult. Most people with AMD have difficulty in low light and at night, and some have difficulty at sundown. See if there is anything in particular the person you live with needs to get done at that time of day, and offer to help.

Simple aids can be the most useful. Depending on the extent of visual loss, you may want to announce your arrival to, and departure from, the room. If you are meeting the person with macular degeneration for lunch or at a museum, try to wear something bright, and provide the person with a description beforehand: "I'll be wearing a yellow jacket." "Look for me—my stocking cap has a bright blue tassel on it." Finding a face in a crowd is very difficult for the person with AMD, but locating you by something you're wearing makes the process much easier. Another idea is, when greeting the person, to state who you are—again, faces can be difficult.

If you're giving the person directions, be clear and use specific terminology. "Turn left" is naturally more helpful than "It's over there."

It is not a faux pas to say to the person, "Did you see the television coverage of the fire?" Making a big deal about the casual use of "see" or any visually related words just makes an issue out of the impairment.

For messages, notes, or letters, use a black felt-tip pen. When writing something on the computer, enlarge the font. If you spend some time with the person, you'll observe how big the lettering should be or how large a font you need to use.

Don't move objects in the person's home. If you use scissors, be sure to put it away, and if you've moved a chair in the den in order to use it somewhere else, put it back. The person with AMD counts on having a predictable environment.

If you're helping with home organization, make certain the person is part of the process. You may think that storing ketchup in the refrigerator door instead of on a shelf makes perfect sense, but the person with the impairment may not be able to find it. Do help with things like tacking down rugs, marking dials, and putting a light-colored liner in the back of dark shelves and cupboards. Those types of chores will be enormously helpful.

If you hand a person with AMD any money, identify what you're giving them. Coins can be recognized by touch, but bills can't, and the person may have difficulty seeing the denomination.

Try to help stave off depression. When the person with AMD gets frustrated trying to learn a new program on the computer, or adjusting a tape recorder, remind her that there are plenty of frustrations in life no matter what you do. Your presence and support will make it easier for the person with AMD.

Helping Someone with Low Vision Get Around

Anyone with AMD should feel free to consult with an orientation and mobility specialist. Those with a serious impairment should have orientation and mobility training, and family members should be involved so that you understand what is helpful and what is not.

Your friend or loved one may need help whenever he is in an unfamiliar location, or maybe just when the lighting is dim, as it is in a movie theater. Tell him that you'd like to help him get around, but only when he needs it.

Once you've had this discussion, try to follow the person with AMD's guidelines as much as possible. No one wants to be treated as if she is incapacitated if she isn't. Of course, you do need to be extra careful if the two of you are in an unusual situation.

When the person does need help, let him take your arm. If you grab his arm, it can throw him off balance. This way he's in control.

If you're walking with someone who's experiencing a great deal of visual difficulty, walk a half step ahead so that your body movements indicate when to change direction, stop, or start, and when to step up or down at a curb. Also provide information as you walk along: "We've just entered the park, and in just a minute we're going to come to three steps that will take us down by the duck pond."

To help someone through a doorway or to begin going down a narrow staircase, move ahead, positioning your guiding arm behind you. With a staircase, be sure the person's hand finds the rail, and give some idea of whether there are a few steps or a longer staircase involved.

To help someone into a car, tell her whether she is getting into the front or the back seat, and place one hand on the car door and the other on the seat back. From there she should be able to seat herself.

Dining Out

If needed, help the person to the table—dim light can make navigating particularly difficult. Place his hands on the chair back once you're there, and let him know if the chair has arms or not and whether or not it is already pulled out from the table. If more than one person is dining with you, indicate who will be to the left and who will be to the right.

People with low vision are often perfectly happy to order the specials that are described by the waiter. Others may use a magnifier to read the menu. However, if you're asked, be prepared to help with the menu.

Once the food comes, knowing what is on the plate can be

difficult for the person with low vision. Again, restaurants are often dim, and the lack of contrast may present a more serious problem than usual. To help with enjoyment of the meal, help the person locate the food by describing it using an imaginary clock as a reference. Vegetables are at six o'clock and the main course is at three o'clock, for example.

Does the person with AMD need help getting to the rest room? In some restaurants the facilities are located on a lower level, which means going down dark staircases. Make certain that your friend or loved one doesn't need verbal guidance or physical assistance.

Remember the Importance of Companionship

The person who is visually impaired almost certainly wants to be independent, but that doesn't mean she wants to be left alone. Think about activities the two of you have always enjoyed doing together, and don't rule out anything without first talking to your friend. Golf, theater, bowling, movies—if your friend used to enjoy these activities, she may still want to participate in them now.

Do the old, but try something new, too. It's important for the person with a visual impairment to feel that there are also new things awaiting him. Anything from a new restaurant to a book club (who said you have to read the book; most popular new books are also out in audio) might hold special enjoyment.

CONCLUSION

What began as a search for answers for my mother has resulted in answers for a condition that may one day affect me. As you have read, I've learned that macular degeneration runs in families, and I know now that my light gray eyes, which pale in comparison to my mother's azure blue ones, are not a sign in my favor.

At the time of her diagnosis, my mother knew more than I did, and her words to me were "Take antioxidant vitamins."

Now I turn to my middle daughter, who inherited her grandmother's stunning blue eyes, and I say, "Wear your dark glasses please, dear." And I mix spinach leaves into all of our salads.

With my "stars marked," so to speak, am I frightened of inheriting macular degeneration? As a writer who loves to read anything and everything, of course the possibility scares me. But then I look at the actress with AMD, the painter, the audio engineer, the business consultant, Dr. Bob Thompson, and my mother, to name just a few, and I see what active and involved lives they are still leading. I hear businessman Max

Cole's words, "Think of what you *can* do, not of what you *can't* do." Life is less convenient for these people, but they have not let their diagnosis inhibit them any more than necessary.

Writing purely as a layperson, I will also note that I believe we are on the cusp of a new age. More money than ever is being devoted to the disease, and though the progress at this point is not conclusive, I think five or ten more years of dedicated research is going to make a big difference.

I can also tell you that I have tried on some amazing devices. Dr. Bob Thompson, who tells his story at the beginning of the book, has profound vision loss, yet on the day that I met him, he moved around the hotel restaurant as if he had full vision. After running back up to the room to bring me some of the low-vision devices, he amazed me by putting on the headset he sometimes wears and describing to me the earring I was wearing. This same headset permitted him to do crossword puzzles on the transatlantic flight to New York from his home in England.

I hate switching reading glasses, so I am the first to acknowledge that there is nothing convenient about reading machines or somewhat cumbersome headsets, but if it's a question of seeing or not seeing, I'll be putting on that headgear.

I'll also think of Dorothy Donovan, age eighty-nine, whose vision loss is now quite severe. She has given up driving but cleans her own home, does her own shopping, listens to books on tape, and when she has to read something, uses a combination of eyeglasses and a magnifying glass, since the cost of a reading machine is beyond her means. Not a hint of self-pity was present during our interview, and we ended our conversation on an upbeat note. Dorothy was very pleased to share something she was eagerly anticipating.

"The other day someone from the Lighthouse asked me if there was anything particular I missed," she told me. "I didn't have to think about it at all before saying, 'I'd like to be able to sew again.' I used to make lots of things—clothing mainly, and things for my home—so I said, 'I'd like to be able to sew.' "

The following week she had an appointment—someone was coming to her home to teach Dorothy how to sew again.

APPENDIX:
WHAT IS COVERED BY INSURANCE
AND WHAT IS NOT

For older adults with vision-impairment, vision-care and vision-rehabilitation therapies are the stepchildren of the Medicare/Medicaid insurance system: very little exists in the way of reimbursement for such services.

If you are experiencing problems with your vision, please visit your regular eye-care practitioner (your ophthalmologist or optometrist). He or she will determine if there is an underlying medical condition or disease and will prescribe or refer you for further medical treatment. If it is determined that your vision cannot be corrected by surgery or with the use of eyeglasses or contact lenses, you may be referred to a low-vision specialist for a low-vision eye examination and evaluation, as described elsewhere in this book.

Refractions, glasses, and low-vision devices may or may not be covered by your insurance. Unfortunately, no universal coverage exists for comprehensive vision-care and vision-rehabilitation services at this time. Some private insurance plans and some government insurance plans, in some places in some states, cover some services and/or devices!

To learn if a low-vision examination is covered by *your* insurance, speak with your doctor or call your insurance plan representative. Call your area agency on aging to find out more about Medicaid benefits in your state and to find out how to reach your state Medicare office. If you do not know or cannot find the phone number for your area agency on aging, call 1-800-677-1116. For more general information about what Medicare covers, call 1-800MEDICARE (1-800-633-4227).

Currently, there is no Medicare coverage under Durable Medical Equipment (DME) for optical devices or low-vision aids, such as a high powered magnifier or a CCTV (closed circuit television). Some success has been achieved, on a case by case basis, in securing reimbursement for the very expensive CCTVs, through a long and arduous appeals process, which is described elsewhere in this book. Call 1-877-HELP WIN for further information.

Without comprehensive coverage for vision-care and vision-rehabilitation services, millions of older adults who could benefit from such services do not have access to them. To begin to shore up this gap, legislation has been introduced in Congress to make orientation and mobility specialists, rehabilitation teachers, and low-vision therapists (see Glossary for definitions of these professionals) eligible providers of services under Medicare. When this bill is passed, the healthcare services furnished by these professionals, to promote the safety and independence of older persons who are blind or partially sighted, will become more available to those Medicare beneficiaries who need them. Additionally, it is hoped that private insurers and Medicaid will follow Medicare's lead and reimburse for the services of these providers as well. To learn more about this pending legislation and how you can help advocate for it, please visit http://www.Medicarenow.org or call 1-877-HELP WIN.

GLOSSARY

Amsler grid. A diagnostic tool that people can use at home to test their own vision for the onset of any distortions caused by AMD. It looks like graph paper with a dot in the middle.

Antiangiogenesis. Angiogenesis is the growth of new blood vessels, and antiangiogenesis is the scientific work being done to find ways to halt the growth of the new, weaker blood vessels that proliferate in macular degeneration. Though it is difficult to reach the retina in a safe, effective manner, scientists hope that an eyedrop or a new technology that permits delivery of a drug to the back of the eye will prove effective.

Antioxidants. Naturally occurring chemicals that assist the body in preventing and arresting some ailments, possibly including macular degeneration. We get antioxidants through eating certain fruits and vegetables; some ophthalmologists and optometrists recommend taking antioxidant vitamin supplements.

Atrophic macular degeneration. The dry form of AMD. More gradual and generally less damaging than the wet form.

Cataract. A clouding of the lens of the eye. People with cataracts see through a haze. In a usually safe and successful surgery, the cloudy lens can be replaced with a plastic lens. AMD is sometimes discovered after a cataract is removed, simply because it is now possible for your eye-care professional to get a better view of the retina. People with AMD should consult with more than one specialist before having a cataract removed, however. Occasionally the removal makes vision worse.

Central vision. Your macula is responsible for central vision, the area of your vision that shows you what is directly in front of you. If you lose central vision, you still have peripheral, or side, vision.

Charles Bonnet syndrome. Approximately 15 percent of people with AMD have occasional hallucinations, and this condition has been dubbed Charles Bonnet syndrome. The hallucinations tend to be unthreatening, and they are not a sign of any type of mental illness. It is thought that CBS is a result of sensory deprivation.

Choroidal neovascularization. Another name for the wet form of AMD.

Closed-circuit television (CCTV). This is not a television; it's a magnifier that looks a bit like a television—or like the microfiche readers at libraries. These devices are reading machines. You can magnify print up to sixty times on them, making them an enormously helpful tool for those with AMD.

Cones. Light-sensitive retinal cells, shaped like cones, that permit sharp vision in bright light. The cones are also responsible for color discrimination.

Disciform macular degeneration. Large scarred area in the retina.

Exudative macular degeneration. The wet form of AMD. Your doctor may write in your charts: "exudative maculopathy."

Fluorescein angiogram. A procedure in which a dye is injected into a patient's bloodstream allowing any abnormal blood vessel hemorrhages in the eye to be seen using a special camera. This test or a similar one is recommended if wet macular degeneration is suspected.

Functional vision. The ability to use your remaining vision, in many instances peripheral vision, to get around.

Hemorrhagic macular degeneration. Wet AMD that involves bleeding in the retina.

Hyperopia. Farsightedness, or a condition in which vision is better for distance than for near objects. Hyperopia is considered a risk factor for AMD because people who are farsighted are less likely to wear glasses much of the time, and even regular glasses offer protection against UV rays.

Indocyanine green angiography (ICG). This test is similar to the fluorescein angiogram and is used to further diagnose wet macular degeneration. In this test, a bright green dye is used for seeing the deeper blood vessels. This dye does contain a form of iodine, so patients allergic to iodine should tell their doctors.

Laser therapy (photocoagulation laser therapy). A treatment in which a beam of light is used to seal leaking blood vessels. Scarring—and a resulting blind spot—often results.

Legal blindness. This is defined as having 20/200 vision in your best eye with correction, or a visual field of 20 degrees or less. This means that with your best eye (wearing glasses or contacts), you see at twenty feet what a normal eye sees at two hundred feet. In addition, your field of vision is only 20 degrees wide rather than the normal 180. Many people who are legally blind still have a great deal of vision left.

Low vision. A visual impairment, not corrected by standard eyeglasses, contact lenses, medication, or surgery, that interferes with the ability to perform everyday activities.

Low-vision specialist. An ophthalmologist or optometrist who specializes in the evaluation of low vision. This person can prescribe visual devices and teach people how to use them.

Low-vision therapist. A person who enables people with vision impairment to enhance the use of their remaining vision for everyday tasks through functional assessments and interventions.

Macula. From the Latin word for "spot," the part of the retina that is responsible for central vision and seeing fine detail.

Myopia. Nearsightedness, or the diminished ability to see objects far away.

Ophthalmologist. A doctor who specializes in eye and vision care and who is trained to provide the full spectrum of eye care, from prescribing medicine and glasses and contact lenses to complex and delicate eye surgery. Many eye M.D.s are also involved in scientific research into the causes and cures for eye diseases and vision problems. Some ophthalmologists have special training in low vision as well.

Optical devices. Prescription and nonprescription devices that help people with low vision enhance their remaining vision. Some examples include magnifiers, telescopic lenses, CCTVs, etc.

Optician. A trained professional who grinds, fits, and dispenses glasses by prescription from an optometrist or ophthalmologist.

Optometrist. A doctor of optometry who examines, diagnoses, treats, and manages diseases and disorders of the eye, as well as diagnoses related systemic conditions. These doctors also prescribe eyeglasses and contact lenses, and medicines to treat eye diseases. An increasing number are also beginning to specialize in low vision, and to diagnose and prescribe low-vision devices and appropriate vision therapy.

Orientation and mobility specialist. A person who teaches people who are visually impaired to move around safely both indoors and outdoors—to learn how to use their residual vision, auditory cues, and/or other mechanisms (white cane, guide dog, human guide) to safely navigate stairs, street corners, busy sidewalks, and public transportation.

Oxidation. A chemical reaction that occurs in the body. Sometimes destructive, as in the case of macular degeneration, it may be facilitated by the energy from light.

Partially sighted. This term refers to someone with a significant reduction of visual function that cannot be corrected to the normal range by ordinary glasses, contact lenses, medical treatment, and/or surgery.

Peripheral vision. The side vision you have out of the corner of your eye. With peripheral vision, you do not see in as much detail as you do with central vision, but you can still see well enough to get around, and with magnification, you can see much more.

Photoreceptors. The rod and cone cells of the retina that absorb the light and let the images come through to the retina (and macula).

Radiation therapy. A form of treatment used to halt the buildup of abnormal blood vessels or other tissues, such as tumors. It has not proven to be as effective in treating AMD as was once hoped.

Rehabilitation teacher. A person who helps people with impaired vision to make lifestyle changes and use alternate techniques to function independently at home, at work, and in the community.

Retina. The layer of tissue that lines the inside of the eye and receives the image formed by the lens.

Retinal specialist. An ophthalmologist who specializes in diseases of the retina. If you've been diagnosed with macular degeneration, you should be checked by a retinal specialist on a regular schedule.

Rods. Light-sensitive retinal cells, shaped like rods, that make it possible to see in dim light and with peripheral vision.

Scotoma(s). A blind spot, which may occur in one's central vision.

Senile macular degeneration. The most commonly used older term for AMD (because it tends to hit an older population).

Stargardt disease. A hereditary form of macular degeneration found in younger people. It is sometimes called juvenile macular degeneration.

Subretinal neovascularization. This happens in wet AMD when vessels grow abnormally and leak in the retina.

Supplements. Vitamin and mineral products intended to add beneficial nutrients that may be missing in someone's diet.

Visual acuity. The ability of the eye to identify objects. Visual acuity is measured by using specially devised charts. The charts are calculated based upon the assumption that the individual is seated twenty feet away from the chart. The top number (numerator) refers to the distance of the chart from the patient; the bottom number (denominator) refers to the distance from which a "normal" person should be able to read the chart. If your distance vision is recorded as 20/200, a person with 20/20 vision can see the same letter at 200 feet.

Visual disability. Also called visual impairment, a condition in which a person lacks enough vision to perform certain tasks.

Vitreous. The clear gel that fills the rear portion of the eyeball, between the lens and the retina.

RESOURCES

Finding Low-Vision Help Locally

Within the text, you've read about how to locate a low-vision clinic or vision-rehabilitation center in your area. However, in some parts of the country what is termed a low-vision center may not offer full service. If you have read about something here that is not offered at your clinic, you can find additional services through your state government. For example, if you need orientation and mobility training or some help in figuring out how to reorganize your home, there are state services that offer such help.

One warning: Change happens slowly, and low vision is just barely being acknowledged as a condition that is very different from being blind. As a result, the resources that will be appropriate and helpful for you may still fall under the umbrella of services for the blind. In reality such services offer help for people with all types of vision deficits.

Each state receives federal funds to run support services for people with visual impairments. The main office will be in the state's capital, so call there first to find a district office near you. (Check the government section of the white pages.) These programs and services differ from state to state. However most include technology training, social services, and/or vocational training.

State technology training centers provide different services in each state. Services may include information and referral services, assistance in obtaining funding for devices and services, demonstrations of adaptive equipment, technology training, equipment exchange, and loan programs.

If you have difficulty locating the proper branch, try contacting the commission on aging in your state or call the toll-free numbers in this section (or call Lighthouse International [800-829-0500]). They'll be able to point you in the right direction. If you're still at a loss, call or visit your local library. A staff member will be able to provide you with the exact information you need.

If you would like help with preparing for employment, contact your state's Department of Rehabilitation for counseling and assistance. Or contact the State Department of Health and Social Services and/or the State Department of Rehabilitation. Most veterans with a visual impairment will be eligible for special services. Contact the VA hospital near you for additional information.

General Information and Referral Services

AMD Alliance International
11460 Johns Creek Parkway
Duluth, GA 30097

hot line: 877-263-7171

http://www.amdalliance.org

American Academy of Ophthalmology
655 Beach St.
San Francisco, CA 94109-7424
415-561-8500

http://www.eyenet.org

For a brochure on AMD, write to Inquiry Clerk—MAC, American Academy of Ophthalmology, P.O. Box 7424, San Francisco, CA 94120-7424.

American Foundation for the Blind
11 Penn Plaza, Suite 300
New York, NY 10001

800-232-5463
212-502-7600

http://www.afb.org

The AFB provides information about services on the national and local level for people who are blind or visually impaired and has offices throughout the United States.

American Optometric Association
243 Lindbergh Blvd.
St. Louis, MO 63141
314-991-4100

http://www.aoanet.org

A low-vision optometrist can be instrumental in helping you see more things clearly. If you can't find a low-vision specialist in your area, contact the American Optometric Association for additional information.

Association for Macular Diseases
210 E. 64th St.
New York, NY 10021

212-605-3719

A national support group that provides a quarterly news-letter to members informing them of new developments regarding macular degeneration. A telephone hotline is available to members. Fee for annual membership dues.

Council of Citizens with Low Vision International
1155 15th St. NW, Suite 1004
Washington, DC 20005

800-733-2258

The Foundation for Fighting Blindness
Executive Plaza 1, Suite 800
11350 McCormick Rd.
Hunt Valley, MD 21031-1014

800-683-5555
410-785-1414

http://www.blindness.org

This organization provides information for all retinal degenerative diseases, including macular degeneration. Some national affiliates have support groups.

International Lions Club
300 W. 22nd St.
Oak Brook, IL 60523

630-571-5466

One of the main interests of the Lions Club organization is helping to give people access to information about vision problems; they also try to provide referrals to low-vision centers.

Lighthouse International

Information and Resource Service
111 E. 59th St.
New York, NY 10022-1202

212-821-9200
800-829-0500
TTY: 212-821-9703

e-mail: info@lighthouse.org
http://www.lighthouse.org

Lighthouse International provides timely information about vision impairment re: eye disorders, vision rehabilitation services, low-vision care, support groups, and resources, including adaptive computer technology, reading and recreation options for people with impaired vision, nutrition, and health.

Macular Degeneration Foundation

P.O. Box 9752
San Jose, CA 95157-9752

408-260-1335

e-mail: eyesight@eyesight.org
http://www.eyesight.org

Nonprofit organization that conducts research and educates patients on various aspects of retinal diseases involved in macular degeneration.

National Association for Visually Handicapped

22 W. 21st St.
New York, NY 10010

212-889-3141

e-mail: staff@navh.org
http://www.navh.org

Serves as a clearinghouse for information about services available to the partially seeing from public and private sources; conducts bicoastal community self-help groups; counsels in the testing and use of visual devices; offers by mail a large-print loan library, newsletters, kits of information, etc.

National Eye Care Project (NECP)
Foundation of the American Academy of Ophthalmology
P.O. Box 429098
San Francisco, CA 94142-9098

800-222-EYES (3937)

National Eye Institute Information Office
Bldg. 31, Room 6A32
31 Center Dr. MSC 2510
Bethesda, MD 20892-2510

301-496-5248

e-mail 2020@nei.nih.gov

Provides publications on eye diseases and information on current eye research.

National Federation of the Blind
1800 Johnson St.
Baltimore, MD 21230

410-659-1443

http://www.nfb.org

Prevent Blindness America
500 E. Remington Rd.
Schaumburg, IL 60173

800-331-2020

e-mail: info@preventblindness.org
http://www.preventblindness.org

Publishes large-print information on AMD, glaucoma, cataracts, etc.; offers toll-free information line, vision screening, and community services through local affiliates and divisions.

Research to Prevent Blindness
645 Madison Ave.
New York, NY 10022-1010

800-621-0026
212-752-4333

http://www.rpbusa.org

Provides free information on all types of eye disease, including the latest in AMD research, plus free visual acuity test cards with the Amsler grid.

Resources for Rehabilitation
33 Bedford St., Suite 19A
Lexington, MA 02420

781-862-6455

e-mail: Info@rfr.org
http://www.rfr.org

Publishes large-print directories such as *Living with Low Vision: A Resource Guide for People with Sight Loss* and *Resources for Elders with Disabilities.*

www.bookmarkets.org

Recorded Reading Materials

American Printing House for the Blind
1839 Frankfort Ave.
P.O. Box 6085
Louisville, KY 40206-0085

800-223-1839
502-895-2405

e-mail: aph@iglou.com
http://www.aph.org

Provides free subscriptions to *Newsweek* and *Reader's Digest* on four-track cassette; catalog also available on cassette, along with two free semiannual catalogs.

Associated Services for the Blind—Recorded Periodicals
919 Walnut St.
Philadelphia, PA 19107

215-627-0600

e-mail: asbinfo@asb.org
http://www.libertynet.net/~asbinfo

Produces braille, tape, and large-print materials for blind and visually impaired persons and the business community.

Books on Tape, Inc.
P.O. Box 7900
Newport Beach, CA 92658-7900

800-626-3333

http://www.booksontape.com

Provides a rental program of full-length books, from classics to best-sellers.

Braille Circulating Library
2700 Stuart Ave.
Richmond, VA 23220-3305

804-359-3743

e-mail: BrailleCl@aol.com

Provides braille and talking books, tapes, cassettes, and large-print materials.

Choice Magazine Listening
85 Channel Dr.
Port Washington, NY 11050-2216

516-883-8280

Offers selected unabridged articles, short stories, and poetry free, bimonthly, from popular print magazines on four-track cassettes. Playable on free special-speed four-track Library of Congress cassette player. Serves college level and older (U.S.)

Educational Tape Recording for the Blind and Disabled, Inc.
3915 W. 103rd St.
Chicago, IL 60655

773-445-3533

Two-track cassettes for students of all ages. $50 annual registration fee.

Library of Congress
National Library Service for the Blind and Physically Handicapped
1291 Taylor St. NW
Washington, DC 20542

800-424-8567
202-707-5100
TDD: 202-707-0744

e-mail: nls@loc.gov
http://lcweb.loc.gov/nls

Administers a national library service that provides braille and recorded books and magazines on free loan to anyone who cannot read standard print because of visual or physical disabilities.

Library Service tapes require a four-track player, which you can borrow from your regional library or purchase. Commercial tapes play back on standard two-track players.

To locate the Libraries for the Blind in your state, call the National Library Service at (800) 424-8567.

Newspapers for the Blind
5508 Calkins Rd.
Flint, MI 48532

810-762-3656

Reads local newspapers over the telephone to subscribers.

Recording for the Blind and Dyslexic
The Anne T. MacDonald Center
20 Roszel Rd.
Princeton, NJ 08540

800-221-4792
609-452-0606
customer service fax: 609-987-8116

http://www.rfbd.org

Lends four-track cassette tapes of books of educational and professional material. Provides direct sale of books on computer disk and specially adapted players and recorders. Registration fee.

Commercial Producers of Books on Tape

Audio Editions
P.O. Box 6930
Auburn, CA 95604

800-231-4261

Books for adults and children. Nonfiction, fiction, self-help.

Audio Renaissance
6 Commerce Way
Arden, NC 28704

800-452-5589

Popular fiction and nonfiction.

Blackstone Audio Books
P.O. Box 969
Ashland, OR 97520

800-729-2665

Unabridged recordings.

Chivers Audio Books
1 Lafayette Rd.
Box 1450
Hampton, NH 03843-1450

800-621-0182

Books for adults and children—audio for adults and children, large print for children only.

Listening Library
One Park Ave.
Old Greenwich, CT 06870-1727

800-243-4504

Books for adults and children.

Recorded Books, Inc.
270 Skip Jack Rd.
Prince Frederick, MD 20678

800-638-1304

Bestsellers and classics.

Large-Print Reading Materials

American Printing House for the Blind
1839 Frankfort Ave.
P.O. Box 6085
Louisville, KY 40206-0085

800-223-1839
502-895-2405

e-mail: aph@iglou.com
http://www.aph.org

Designated by Congress as the official source of textbooks for students who are visually impaired, and maintains a centralized database of large print. Provides large-type textbooks, cookbooks, dictionaries, etc. Catalog available on request.

Blindskills, Inc.
P.O. Box 5181
Salem, OR 97304-0181

800-860-4224
503-581-4224

e-mail: blindskl@teleport.com

Publishes a quarterly magazine in large print, braille, and four-track cassette.

Doubleday Large Print Home Library
Membership Services Center
6550 E. 30th St.
P.O. Box 6325
Indianapolis, IN 46206

317-541-8920 (dial "O" for operator)

Provides hardcover editions of bestsellers in large print, cassette music tapes, and videos.

G.K. Hall and Co.
Gale Group
P.O. Box 9187
Farmington Hills, MI 48331

248-699-4253

http://www.mlr.com/thorndike

Provides direct sale of large-print books.

ISIS Large Print Books
Transaction Publishers
Rutgers University
New Brunswick, NJ 08903

732-445-2280
732-932-2280

Literature, biography, and reference.

New York Times/Large Type Weekly
229 W. 43rd St.
New York, NY 10036

800-631-2580

Weekly edition of the *New York Times* in large print.

Reader's Digest Large-Type Edition for Easier Reading
P.O. Box 3010
Harlan, IA 51593

800-807-2780

http: www.readersdigest.com

Offers subscription to large-type edition of *Reader's Digest* magazine; nonglare paper.

Reader's Digest Large-Type Reader
P.O. Box 3010
Harlan, IA 51593

800-877-5293

Offers yearly, six-volume subscriptions of choice reading from Reader's Digest Select Editions.

Ulverscroft Large Print (USA), Inc.
P.O. Box 1230
West Seneca, NY 14224-1230

800-955-9659

e-mail: sales@ulverscroftusa.com
http://www.ulverscroft.co.uk

Provides direct sale of large-print books—mystery, romance, classic literature, and nonfiction.

Optical Reading and Illumination Devices

Consult with a low-vision specialist before making final selection of these items.

Bossert Specialties
3620 E. Thomas Rd., Suite D-124
Phoenix, AZ 85018

800-776-5885

http://bossertspecialties.com

Specializes in products for the visually impaired, such as visual aid devices, accessories, and software. Offers a catalog and online specialty store.

Lighthouse International
111 E. 59th St.
New York, NY 10022-1202

800-829-0500

e-mail: lighthousecatalog@lighthouse.org

59th Street (NYC) store offers wide variety of products, which are also featured in the catalog.

Materials Center
National Federation of the Blind
1800 Johnson St.
Baltimore, MD 21230

410-659-9314

http://www.nfb.org

Publications on Adaptive Technology

AccessWorld, a new publication, is now available from the American Foundation for the Blind, and promises to be a comprehensive resource for obtaining the latest information on adaptive technology and visual impairment. Written for the layperson, the magazine promises product evaluations, new product announcements, information on the latest developments in the field, and feedback from readers. $29.95 for six issues. Contact:

AccessWorld/AFB Press
Subscription Services
450 Fame Ave.
Hanover, PA 17331

Or order by calling 888-522-0220 or faxing 717-633-8920

http://www.afb.org/accessworld

Support Groups and Consumer-Related Organizations

AARP
601 E St. NW
Washington, DC 20049

800-424-3410

http://www.aarp.org

Association of Driver Educators for the Diabled
P.O. Box 49
Edgerton, WI 53534

608-884-8833

Lighthouse International
111 E. 59th St.
New York, NY 10022-1202

800-829-0500

e-mail: info@lighthouse.org
http://www.lighthouse.org

Provides all types of resources and support for people who are visually impaired. Lighthouse International is a not-for-profit organization that relies on the support and generosity of individuals, foundations, and organizations.

National Association for the Visually Handicapped
22 W. 21 St.
New York, NY 10010

212-889-3141

e-mail: staff@navh.org
http://www.navh.org

Offers support groups and guides others on how to form such groups.

National Association of Professional Organizers
P.O. Box 140647
Austin, TX 78714

Referral Line: 512-206-0151

Religious Resources

American Bible Society
1865 Broadway
New York, NY 10023

212-408-1200

http://www.americanbible.org

Aurora Ministries
P.O. Box 621
Bradenton, FL 34206

941-748-3031

Offers recorded scriptures in fifty-two languages on cassette tapes free to the blind, visually impaired, and print handicapped. (Verification of impairment required.)

Christian Record Services, Inc.
4444 S. 52nd St.
Lincoln, NE 68516

Mailing address:
P.O. Box 6097
Lincoln, NE 68506

402-488-0981

e-mail: CRSnet@compuserve.com
http://www.ChristianRecord.org

Provides free Christian publications and programs for people with visual impairments.

Jewish Braille Institute of America
110 E. 30th St.
New York, NY 10016

212-889-2525
800-433-1531

e-mail: admin@jewishbraille.org
http://www.jewishbraille.org

Provides a broad variety of Jewish reading materials in braille, large print, and talking books and serves people in nearly fifty countries through its multilingual resources.

John Milton Society for the Blind
475 Riverside Dr., Room 455
New York, NY 10115

212-870-3336

e-mail: order@jmsblind.org
http://www.jmsblind.org

Provides free religious and inspirational materials.

Walker and Company
435 Hudson St.
New York, NY 10014

212-727-8300

Large-print books on Judaism and Christianity.

Xavier Society for the Blind
154 E. 23rd St.
New York, NY 10010-4595

800-637-9193
212-473-7800

Religious and inspirational material in braille, large print, and on tape.

Radio Reading

Radio reading services broadcast recordings of periodicals and daily newspapers over special channels. To find a service near you call:

In Touch Networks, Inc.
15 W. 65th St.
New York, NY 10023

212-769-6270

Newsline for the Blind

A computerized newspaper reading service developed by the National Federation of the Blind. Users call a special phone number to listen to free computerized readings of *USA Today*, the *New York Times*, and the *Chicago Tribune*. The service is currently available in over thirty-five cities and growing constantly.

National Federation of the Blind
1800 Johnson St.
Baltimore, MD 21230

410-659-9314

http://www.nfb.org

Audio Description

Many television programs and videos are now available with narration of key visual elements and action. For more information:

Descriptive Video Service
WGBH (DVS)
125 Western Ave.
Boston, MA 02134

800-333-1203
617-300-3490

www.wgbh.org/dvs

Nostalgia Good TV
650 Massachusetts Ave., NW
Washington, DC 20001

202-562-0044

Machines That Read Text Aloud

Personal readers scan printed material and translate it into simulated human speech. Some companies that make personal readers are

Arkenstone
Nasa Ames Mossett Complex
P.O. Box 215
Mossettfield, CA 94035

650-603-8880
800-444-4443

Kurzweil
52 Third Ave.
Burlington, MA 01803

781-203-5000
800-894-5374

Closed-Circuit Televisions

Closed-circuit televisions (CCTVs) help many people who have low vision to read books, newspapers, and correspondence by displaying a magnified image of text on a video monitor. Demonstrations can be arranged, and while the machines are expensive, monthly payment plans are available. Some of the machines offer several options to improve the viewing of printed material (high-contrast full color, full-color photo, yellow letters on black background, green letters on blue background, amber letters on black background, and white text on black—ideal for reading text because there is less glare). Even with all these options, companies have tried to keep operating units simple so that an on/off switch, a lever that sets magnification level, a control that adjusts background, and a focus knob are the only controls that need to be set—very easy when you're actually sitting in front of a machine. Anything from an encyclopedia to a postcard can be viewed on one of these, and some people use them for enhanced viewing while doing tasks such as check writing.

Closed-circuit televisions are a major expense—and they are well worth the investment if you really need one—but you don't want to be talked into spending the money needlessly. That's why it's important to speak with your low-vision specialist to be certain there isn't a less costly solution.

Internet Portals

LighthouseLink

http//:www.lighthouselink.org

"LighthouseLink" is a fully accessible, interactive not-for-profit site providing helpful information to people who are visually impaired and their families as well as linking them to a wide variety of resources on the Internet. LighthouseLink is sponsored by Lighthouse International in partnership with not-for-profit agencies worldwide.

We Media

http://www.wemedia.com

We Media, a relatively young company serving the disabled and their families, recently unveiled a full-service Web site aimed at that market. While it appears to be like most other commercial or service sites, with lots of information and links to shopping, each mouse click also leads to a wide range of offerings (educational, employment, real estate, travel, financial services) that are geared to the needs of the disabled. The site also offers users free e-mail and computer-based long-distance calls over the Internet. Portions of the site, like *We Media* magazine, also have special software that enables users with impaired vision to hear rather than read, and they report that they are making aggressive efforts to make the site totally accessible.

Large-Print Music

Large-Print Music is a new series of piano and vocal sheet music for people who are visually impaired. Selections include pop standards, hymns, and various classical piano selections.

Stephens Development Co.
3542 Fair Oaks Lane
Longboat Key, FL 34228

941-383-4398

Catalogs of Helpful Products

Contact each of these companies and ask for a catalog. You'll be stunned at the number of products available to you. (A marked-up catalog will provide family members with plenty of hints about what you'd like for your birthday!)

Ann Morris Enterprises
890 Fams Court
East Meadow, NY 11554-5101

800-454-3175
Fax orders: 516-564-9692

Independent Living Aids
27 E. Mall
Plainview, NY 11803

1-800-537-2118
Fax orders: 516-752-3135

e-mail: indlivaids@aol.com
http://www.independentliving.com

The Lighthouse Catalog
111 E. 59 St.
12th Floor
New York, NY 10022-1202

800-829-0500
Fax orders: 212-821-9727
Or order online: http://www.lighthouse.org

LS&S Group
P.O. Box 673
Northbrook, IL 60065

Information: 847-498-9777
Phone orders: 800-468-4789
Fax orders: 847-498-1482

http://www.lssgroup.com

Maxi-Aids
P.O. Box 3209
Farmingdale, NY 11735

800-522-6294
Fax orders: 1-516-752-0689

National Federation of the Blind
Materials Center
1800 Johnson St.
Baltimore, MD 21230

410-659-9314

http://www.nfb.org/aids&a99.htm

Science Products
P.O. Box 888
Southeastern, PA 19399

800-888-7400

ACKNOWLEDGMENTS

Many people deserve special recognition for the time they devoted to helping us with the preparation of this book. Dr. Barbara Silverstone and the dedicated Vision Rehabilitation, Education, and Research staff of Lighthouse International are worthy of thanks for all that they have done and are continuing to do to further research and rehabilitation for people managing all types of visual difficulties. We appreciate all the information that was shared with us as we worked on the book. Special appreciation is also due to Dr. Eleanor E. Faye, who has led the way in the field of low vision and has affected so much of the work in this area. Thanks also to the gifted Lighthouse International staff members who have helped us: Dr. Amy Horowitz, Dr. Aries Arditi, Nancy Paskin, Martin Yablonski, Dr. Kent Higgins, Karen Seidman, Cathy Czeto, Cynthia Stuen, and Mary Ann Lang. Fran Freedman and Lorraine Lidoff are to be commended for their legislative efforts to benefit the consumer, as is the Communications staff for their tireless efforts trying to educate the public about low vision and macular degeneration, especially during Lighthouse International–inspired National Vision Rehabilitation Day.

Thanks to the Board of the AMD Macular Alliance International, especially Dr. Bob Thompson, Chair of the Executive Committee and an inspiration to many, and to Kelly C. Johnson, Courtney Perry of Ketchum, Jim Harris, Kathrin Wyss, and Christoph Lorez of CIBA/Novartis, who have worked on heightening the awareness and treatment of AMD.

Retinal specialists Drs. Lawrence Yannuzzi, David Guyer, K. Bailey Freund, Jason Slakter, Keith Zinn, Stanley Chang have brought the treatment of macular degeneration into the 21st century.

Chuck Hess, low-vision driving expert, offered invaluable information for the chapter on driving. We also would like to thank Lori L. Grover, OD, FAAO, and Terra Barnes, OD, FAAO, for their efforts in gathering all the state-by-state information that affects low-vision drivers.

Dr. Stuart P. Richer was instrumental in advising us on the chapter concerning nutrition and its affect on macular degeneration. He continues to work hard to conduct studies that will lead to even more definitive information.

Dr. Stanley Wainapel, clinical director of rehabilitation medicine at Montefiore Hospital, and Dr. Lisa Weiss deserve thanks for their help in devising strategies for managing the emotional aspects of macular degeneration.

A very special recognition to a few of the dynamic low-vision clinicians who continue to provide clinical care, educate, write, and work for the benefit of their patients: Drs. Roy G. Cole, Jay M. Cohen, Michael Fischer, Paul and Kathy Freeman, Susan Gormezano, William O'Connell, Wayne Hoeft, Randy Jose, Mary Beth Schanz, Larry Spitzberg, and Tracy Williams.

To the pioneers: Drs. Robert Rosenberg, Al Rosenbloom, and George Hellinger.

Thanks also to the designers and manufacturers who have made living with AMD much easier: Richard Feinbloom of Designs for Vision, Dr. Henry Greene of Ocutech, Jeff Moss of Eschenbach, Ed Bettinardi and Tom Winter of Innoventions, Dave Kerko and Betty Lou Taynton of Corning Medical Optics, Brooks Gleichert of NOIR, Bill Mattingly of Lighthouse International, and John Newt of COIL.

We would also like to mention Bruce's clinical colleagues, who have worked tirelessly in low vision for the past thirty years. Special recognition to the Low Vision Diplomates of the American Academy of Optometry, the 700+ strong members of the Low Vision Section of the American Optometric Association, and those members of the Low Vision Committee of the American Academy of Ophthalmology who are working to unify the low vision field.

We also owe our gratitude to our editor, Ellen Edwards, who worked tirelessly to be certain that the book was the best that it could be. Assisting her at NAL was John Paine, who made certain that all the information was presented as clearly as possible. Thanks, too, to agent Judith Riven, who believed from the beginning that this could be a helpful book.

Dr. Bruce P. Rosenthal
Kate Kelly
April 2001

INDEX

Activities of daily living, 5
  accomplishing a task, 159–160
  calendar and to-do list, 151–152
  check signing, 155–157
  eating, 157–158
  evaluation of, 43–44
  finding a dropped/missing item, 160–162
  folding money, 154–155
  food/liquid handling, 157–158
  paying bills, 155
  personal grooming, 159
  reminder notebook, 152
  sense of humor, 162
  telephone, 152–153
  writing by hand, 155–157
Age-related macular degeneration (AMD), 3
  coping with diagnosis, 19–21, 46–49
  diet/nutrition, 46, 75–85
  driving, 163–193
  explaining condition to others, 50–52
  gathering information, 11, 14, 19–21,
    39–41, 54
  getting around, 48–49, 89–102, 194–222
  helping someone with AMD, 217–218
  keeping current on studies and treatment,
    11, 14, 21, 54
  keeping track of your condition, 41–42
  living well, 131–140, 215–217
  low-vision devices, 103–128
  maximizing sight, 89–102
  pathological process to the eye, 24–34
  questions to ask, 39–41
  risk factors, 67–74
  seeing better, 90–93, 195
  seeking best advice, 42–44
  social contact, 203–205
  treatment options, 53–66
  types. See Dry macular degeneration; Wet
    macular degeneration
  working with your doctor/eye-care team,
    7, 22–23, 36–44, 63–66, 72–74
Aging population:
  AMD risk factor, 67–68
  risk for macular degeneration, 3
AMD Alliance International, 4–5, 7–12, 54
American Academy of Ophthalmology, 43,
  69
American Heart Association, 79
American Optometric Association, 43
Amsler grid, 36–37, 57, 72
Angiostatic steroid injection, 14
Anterior segment specialist, 32
Antioxidants, 3, 72, 76–77
Anti-VEGF therapy, 14
Art galleries, 208–209
Atrophic macular degeneration. See Dry
  macular degeneration
Automobiles, driving of. See Driving

Bathroom safety, 148–149
Bilberry, 83
Blindness:
  legally blind, 19, 33–34
  partial vision with AMD, 19

Blind spot, 90
  after laser surgery, 57
  seeing around, 44
Blood-thinners, 41
Blood vessel growth in wet AMD, 7, 8, 13
Books on tape, 2, 101–102
Borge, Victor, 111, 124
Braille, 20
Bright acuity tester, 45

Cars, driving of. *See Driving*
Cataracts, 31–32, 72, 85
Central vision, changes with AMD, 8, 31,
    32–33
Changes with AMD:
  diet/nutrition, 46, 75–85
  driving, 163–193
  eyes, changes with AMD, 23–34, 49–50
  home/household, 93–99, 132–150
  independence, 131–140, 163–193,
    200–222
  See also Lifestyle changes
Charles Bonnet syndrome, 49–50
Choroidal neovascularization, 30
Choroidal new vessels (CNVs) in wet AMD,
    30
Chromalux lightbulbs, 96
Clinical trials and eligibility, 63–66
Closed-circuit televisions (CCTV),
    111–114
Clutter, clearing of, 133–134
Color of eyes, AMD risk factor, 68, 77
Color perception:
  changes with AMD, 35
  normal changes with age, 28
Commission for the Blind, 34, 43, 132
Commission on the Aging, 132
Common worries about AMD, 19–21
Computer-enhanced indocyanine green
    video angiography (ICG), 38
Computers:
  adapters, 11
  vision devices, 117–119
Contrast sensitivity, 45
Coping with AMD, 46–49, 213–215
Cornea, changes with AMD, 25
Counseling, 43, 214–215

Daily activities. *See Activities of daily living*
Depression, 9, 46, 47, 213–215
Depth perception, 35
Detecting AMD, 36–38
Diet/nutrition, 46, 75–85
  antioxidants, 3, 72, 76–77

bilberry, 83
foods for healthy diet, 79–81
heart healthy diet, 70, 75–85
herbal supplements, 83
high-fat diet/high cholesterol, 70
lutein, 72, 77–78
making changes, 81–82
supplements, 82–84
vegetables, 76–82
vitamins/supplements, 76–84
zeaxanthin, 72, 77–78
zinc, 83–84
Dining out, 218–219
Diopter, 108–109, 122
Disease process of AMD, 23–34
Doctor/eye-care professionals:
  getting a second opinion, 39–40
  keeping track of your condition, 41–42
  questions to ask, 39–41
  reviewing of all medications, 41, 84
  your team of professionals, 22–23
Driving, 163–193
  AARP mature driving course, 178–179
  avoiding accidents, 186
  bad weather, 182–183
  bioptic glasses with restricted license,
    166–178
  car safety, 179–181
  daytime lights, 184
  deciding to stop driving, 187–189
  distractions, 183
  finding your blind spot, 180
  glare, 180
  hearing/reaction time, 185
  license renewal, 164–166
  night driving, 181–182
  others do the driving, 192–193
  other transportation, 189–190
  public transportation, 189, 190–191
  restricted license, 166
  rush hour, 182–183
  safe driving, 183–184
  sunrise/sunset glare, 182–183
  taxis/contract drivers, 191–192
Drugs:
  angiostatic steroid injection, 14
  caution with blood thinners, 41
  clinical trials, 14
  eligibility for clinical trials, 63–66
  metalloproteinase inhibitors, 14
  reviewing all medications with doctor, 41,
    84
  Visudyne, 13
Drusen, 29–30, 36

Dry macular degeneration, 7, 8
  atrophic macular degeneration, 29
  deterioration of central vision, 8
  diet/nutrition study, 78–79
  drusen under retina, 29–30
  laser treatment for drusen, 60–61
  percentage of legally blind, 8
  preventing progression to wet AMD, 13
  progression to wet AMD, 30
  proliferation of weak blood vessels, 30
  questions to ask the doctor, 39–41
  signs of, 29–30
  treatment options, 53
Durable medical equipment, Medicare
    coverage of, 124–126

Eccentric viewing, 90–91
Electronic books, 100–101
Emergency measures in the home, 143–144,
    145
Exercise, 70, 75, 205–206
Eye-care/vision team of professionals, 22–23
Eye examination, detecting AMD, 35–38
Eyes:
  burning, 28
  dryness, 28
  examination of, 35–38
  eye color, AMD risk factor, 68, 77
  fatigue, 28
  floaters, 28
  normal changes with age, 27–28
  normal loss of contrast, 28
  sandy feeling, 28
  self-monitoring condition, 72
  vision distortion, 24–25
  vitreous gel floaters, 28
  wearing eyes out, 20
Eyes, changes with AMD:
  Charles Bonnet syndrome, 49–50
  contrast sensitivity, 45
  cornea, 25
  destruction of retinal pigment epithelium
    (RPE), 28–29
  disease process of AMD, 23–34
  fovea, 27
  glare management, 45
  hallucinations, 49–50
  iris and pupil, 25
  lens and vitreous gel, 26
  macula, 26–27
  macular degeneration, 28–29
  macular pigment density, 45–46
  optic nerve, 25
  photoreceptor cells, 26, 27

  retina, 26
  retinal pigment epithelium (RPE), 26, 27,
    28–29
  rods and cones, 27, 28–29
  "rusting" of macular degeneration, 28–29
  visual changes, 24, 26, 27

Farsightedness, AMD risk factor, 69
Faye, Eleanor, 73–74, 84
FDA. See Food and Drug Administration
    (FDA)
Fire safety in home, 143–144
Floaters, normal changes in eye, 28
Fluorescein angiography, 38, 57
Fluorescent lightbulbs, 95–96
Folding money, 154–155
Font size, 100
Food and Drug Administration (FDA):
  laser cataract surgery, 32
  Optrin priority review, 56
  PDT approval, 54–55
  photodynamic therapy, 13
  PhotoPoint SnET2 priority review, 56
  priority studies, 55–56
  researching clinical trials, 65–66
  Visudyne approval, 55
  Visudyne photodynamic therapy, 13
Food/diet. See Diet/nutrition
Fovea, changes with AMD, 27
Friendship and companionship, 219
Functional vision, 33

Gender, AMD risk factor, 68
Genetics, AMD risk factor, 68–69
Glare, 97–98
  hats and visors, 97–98
  sensitivity testing, 45
  sunglasses, 97
Glasses, 20
  anti-glare sunglasses, 97
  anti-reflective coating, 92
  correct prescription, 41
  dark glasses, 44
  double-checking prescription, 92–93
  sunglasses, 71–73
  tinted, 92
Grieving losses, 11
Grocery shopping, 200–203
  See also Diet/nutrition
Grunwald, Henry, 20–21, 51
Guyer, David, 5, 13–14, 61

Hallucinations with AMD, 49–50
Halogen lighting, 96

Harvard Medical School, nutrition/diet study, 82
Head-mounted video aid, 10
Hearing difficulty with AMD, 205
Herbal supplements, 83
High blood pressure, link with AMD, 70–71
High-fat diet/high cholesterol, AMD risk factor, 70
Hobbies, 209
Home/household:
　bathroom safety, 148–149
　clearing clutter, 133–134
　clocks, 98
　closet organization, 149–150
　contrasting objects, 99, 146
　fire safety, 143–144
　furniture placement, 143
　games in large type, 99
　in the kitchen, 2, 3, 10, 143–148, 157–158
　large-type items, 98, 99
　lighting, 10, 93–97
　living well, 131–140
　low-vision products, 137–138
　magnifying mirrors, 98
　marking and labeling, 136–137
　modified appliances, 98–99
　navigating, 142–143
　organizing, 132–138
　peripheral vision features, 98–99
　place for everything, 134–136
　rearranging rooms, 10
　safety/emergency measures, 143–144, 145
　small recorder for managing projects, 98
　smoke alarms, 143–144
　stairs/steps, 143
　TV/VCR remote control, 98
　visible dials, 146–147
Horowitz, Amy, 47, 49, 213

Illumination/lighting, 93–97
Incandescent lightbulbs, 95
Independence:
　adjusting to new life, 139–140
　advice for those helping, 212–222
　driving, 163–193
　educating others about AMD, 204–205
　friendship and companionship, 219
　help from others, 138
　learning curve and practice, 139–140
　living well, 131–140
　maintaining lifestyle, 18
　recognizing faces, 17, 35, 51, 204
　shopping for clothes, 203
　shopping for groceries, 200–203

social contact, 203–205
Internet conversion programs visual aid, 119
Iris and pupil, changes with AMD, 25

Jordy video headset, 116

Kitchen:
　appliances, 147–148
　contrasting objects, 146
　eating, 157–158
　food/liquid handling, 157–158
　lighting, 10
　measuring, 147
　oven dial marking, 2
　reading recipes, 3
　See also Home/household

Lamps/lighting, 93–97
Laser treatment:
　cool laser in photodynamic therapy (PDT), 54–55
　for drusen in dry macular degeneration, 60–61
　hot laser, 8
　laser cataract surgery, 32
　laser-induced retinal damage, 13
　photocoagulation laser therapy, 56–58
Legal blindness, 7, 33–34
　common worries, 19
　talking book services, 101–102
Lens and vitreous gel, changes with AMD, 26
Library of Congress National Library Services Talking Book Program, 101–102
Lifestyle changes:
　adjusting to new life, 139–140
　daily activities, 43–44, 151–162
　diet/nutrition, 3, 46, 75–85
　driving, 163–193
　independence, 18, 131–140, 163–193, 200–222
　learning curve and practice, 139–140
　living well, 131–140, 215–217
　social contact, 17, 35, 51, 203–205
Light eye color, AMD risk factor, 68, 77
Lighthouse International:
　depression study, 47
　financial assistance for low-vision devices, 124, 125
　full-service vision-rehabilitation center, 42–43
　Low Vision Programs, 3
　rehabilitation teaching, 132

Lighthouse International *(cont'd)*
  researching clinical trials, 64
  survey of vision impairment, 17–18
  volunteers for reading, 102
  Web site, 54
Lighting, 10, 93–97
  adjustment changes with age, 27–28
  managing glare, 97–98
  types of bulbs and lamps, 95–96
Lions Club, 43, 124
Losses with AMD:
  center vision, 8
  driving a car, 9, 17
  independence, 9
  reading, 17
  recognizing faces, 17, 35, 51, 204
Low vision:
  description of, 34
  evaluating your needs, 43–44
  products and devices, 137–138
Low-vision devices, 10, 103–128
  closed-circuit televisions (CCTV),
    111–114
  computers, 117–119
  computer screen magnification, 118
  diopter, 108–109, 122
  evaluating your needs, 121–122
  frame-mounted binoculars, 11
  future technologies, 126–128
  hand and stand magnifiers, 106–107
  Internet conversion programs, 119
  looking normal, 124
  Low Vision Enhancement System
    (LVES), 115–116
  magnification devices, 104, 105–111
  magnifying spectacles, 107–110
  Medicare coverage of, 124–126
  nonoptical devices, 140
  optical character recognition machines
    (OCR), 117
  paying for devices, 124–126
  practicing with device, 122–124
  reading machines, 111–114
  reading materials, 99–102
  relative distance magnification, 103, 104
  relative size magnification, 103–104
  selecting appropriate devices, 119–122
  telescopes and telescopic lenses, 110–111,
    112
  text-to-speech and speech-to-text
    software, 118–119
  training for, 119–120
  video headsets, 115–116
  wearable computers, 127

working with remaining vision, 20–21
Low-vision programs:
  College of Optometry, New York, 4
  Lighthouse International, 3, 4
Low-vision specialist, 22–23, 42
Lutein, 72, 77–78

Macula:
  changes with AMD, 26–27
  macular pigment density, 45–46
  macular translocation surgery, 60
Macular degeneration:
  age-related, 3
  process of, 28–29
Magnification:
  angular magnification, 103, 104
  relative distance, 103, 104
  relative size, 103–104
Magnification devices:
  diopter, 108–109, 122
  hand and stand magnifiers, 106–107
  high-plus spectacles, 107–110
  magnifying spectacles, 107–110
  microscopic lenses, 107–110
  telescopes and telescopic lenses, 110–111,
    112
Magnifying glass, 2
Makeup, application of, 159
Marking and labeling in household, 136–137
Medicare:
  appeal process for low-vision device
    coverage, 125–126
  coverage for vision-rehabilitation services,
    5
  HCFA FORM 1490, 125
  reconsideration of denial, 126
Medications:
  caution with blood thinners, 41
  clinical trials for AMD treatment, 61–62
  marking and labeling, 153–154
  reviewing all drugs with doctor, 41, 84
Menopause, AMD risk, 77
Metalloproteinase inhibitors, 14
Microcurrent stimulation (MCS), 62
Money, handling, 54–55
Museums, 208–209

National Association of Family Services, 215
National Association of Professional
    Organizers, 134
National Eye Institute:
  Age Related Eye Disease Study, 77
  awareness campaign, 18
  diet/nutrition study, 84–85

research, 54
researching clinical trials, 64
submacular surgery trials, 59
Navigating on foot, 194–200
NuVision video headset, 116

Occupational therapists, 23
Ophthalmic nurses, 23
Ophthalmologist, 22
Optical character recognition machines (OCR), 117
Optician, 22
Optic nerve, changes with AMD, 25
Optometrist, 22
Organizing the household, 132–138
Orientation-mobility specialist, 23, 127

Paskin, Nancy, 132, 159
Pathological process of AMD, 24–34
Peripheral vision, 17, 32–33
low-vision devices, 19
seeing around blind spot, 90
training, 11
Personal grooming, 159
Pharmaceutical research:
AE-941 clinical trial, 61
anti-VEGF (vascular endothelial growth factor), 61
pigment epithelium-derived factor, 61
research for AMD treatment, 53
Photocoagulation laser therapy, 56–58
Photodynamic therapy (PDT), 54–55
Photoreceptor cells, changes with AMD, 26, 27
Prevent Blindness America, 18
Protective eyewear, 71–73, 75
Proton therapy, 62
Psychological trauma with AMD diagnosis, 9
Psychologist, counseling with, 43

Questions to ask the doctor/eye care professional, 39–41

Race, AMD risk factor, 68
Radiation therapy, 58
Reading:
books on tape, 101–102
difficulties with, 17, 35
electronic books, 100–101
font size, 100
large-print magazines, 100
low-vision devices, 19
materials for low vision, 12, 99–102

talking book services, 101–102
typoscope, 101
Reading machines, 111–114
Recognizing faces, 17, 35, 51, 204
Rehabilitation teachers, 23
Research:
government funding, 18, 21
National Eye Institute, 54
pharmaceutical studies, 21, 53, 61
Retina:
altered pigment, 36
atrophy of RPE, 36
changes with AMD, 26
keeping track of your condition, 41–42
submacular surgery, 58–59
Retinal pigment epithelium (RPE):
atrophy of, 36
cell transplantation, 59–60
changes with AMD, 26, 27
Retinal specialist, 22, 38
Rheotherapy, 62–63
Richer, Stuart, 78
Risk factors:
age, 67–68
AMD in one eye, 69
circulation, 70–71
farsightedness, 69
gender, 68
genetics, 68–69
light eye color, 68
link with high blood pressure, 70–71
race, 68
self-monitoring, 72–74
smoking, 3, 69–70
sun exposure, 71–72
Rods and cones, changes with AMD, 27
Rosenthal, Bruce, 3–4

Sadness and loss, 11, 46–49
Safety:
in the bathroom, 148–149
driving, 179–181
emergency measures, 143–144, 145
fire safety in home, 143–144
in the kitchen, 144–145
Scanning, 91–92, 195
Scotoma, 44, 90
Seeing better:
blind spot/scotoma, 90
eccentric viewing, 90–91
eyeglasses, 92–93
lighting, 93–97
scanning, 91–92, 195
Self-help groups, 12

Sense of humor, 162, 205
Shaving, 159
Shopping, 200–203
Smoking, AMD risk factor, 69–70, 75, 77
Social contact, 203–205
Social Security, benefits for legal blindness, 34
Social situations:
    appearing aloof, 51
    recognizing faces, 17, 35, 51, 204
Social worker, counseling with, 43
Sports, 207–208
Submacular surgery, 58–59
Subnormal vision. *See low vision*
Sun exposure, AMD risk factor, 71–72
Supplements to diet, 76–84

Telephone/telephone books, 11, 152–153
Telescopes and telescopic lenses, 110–111, 112
Television, viewing aids, 2, 98
Text-to-speech and speech-to-text software, 118–119
Theater, 208
Thompson, Bob, 4–5, 7–12
Total blindness, 19
Tracing while walking, 195–196
Transpupillary Thermotherapy (TTT), 58
Treatment options, 14, 53–66
Twilight: Losing Sight, Gaining Insight (Grunwald), 20–21, 51
Typoscopes, 101

Vegetables, 76–82
Video headsets, 115–116
Vision:
    central vision, 8, 31, 32–33
    distortion with AMD, 24–25
    functional vision, 33
    legal blindness, 7, 19, 33–34, 101–102
    low vision, 34, 43–44
    low-vision evaluation and prescription, 103
    macular vision, 32–33
    peripheral vision, 11, 17, 19, 32–33, 90
    self-monitoring, 72
    visual acuity, 33
Vision care team of professionals, 22–23
Vision-rehabilitation center:
    features of full-service center, 43
    finding one, 42–43
Vision-rehabilitation therapists, 23, 43, 131–140
Visual acuity, 33, 41, 61
    driving license renewal, 164–165
Visual field, driving license renewal, 164–165

Visudyne treatment, 55
Vitamins, 3, 72, 76–77, 76–83
V-Max vision enhancement system, 115–116
Volunteer work, 209–211

Wainapel, Stanley, 47
Walking/navigating on foot:
    grocery shopping, 200–203
    guide dog, 198, 199
    handheld magnifier, 200
    hearing, 196
    pocket flashlight, 199–200
    public spaces, 200
    scanning during walking, 195–196
    shopping for clothes, 203
    spotting, 196
    streets/street systems, 197–198
    telescopic vision aid, 199
    tracing while walking, 195–196
    tracking, 196
    white cane, 198–199
Web sites:
    AMD Alliance International, 54
    Lighthouse International, 54
    See also Resources
Weiss, Lisa, 46, 48, 215
Wet macular degeneration, 7–8
    abnormal blood vessel growth or bleeding, 14
    Amsler grid, 36–37, 57, 72
    choroidal neovascularization, 30
    choroidal new vessels (CNVs), 30
    computer-enhanced indocyanine green video angiography (ICG), 38
    early symptoms, 30–31
    fluorescein angiography, 38
    legally blind status, 30
    photocoagulation laser therapy, 56–58
    photodynamic therapy (PDT), 54–55
    proton therapy trial, 62
    questions to ask the doctor, 39–41
    radiation therapy, 58
    rapid loss of central vision, 31
    retinal distortion or scar tissue, 30
    Transpupillary Thermotherapy (TTT), 58
    treatment options, 53
Wilmer Ophthalmological Institute, 50
Writing:
    checks, 155–157
    by hand, 155–157
    letters, 11

Zeaxanthin, 72, 77–78
Zinc, 83–84